The Presence
of Caring in Nursing

Delores A. Gaut
Editor

National League for Nursing Press • New York
Pub. No. 15-2465

The Presence of
Caring in Nursing

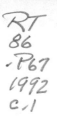

#25828642

The views expressed in this publication represent the views of the authors and do not neccessarily reflect the official views of the National League for Nursing Press.

This book was set in Goudy by Publications Development Company. The editor and designer was Allan Graubard. Northeastern Press was the printer and binder. The cover was designed by Lillian Welsh.

Printed in the United States of America

Contents

Contributors

Mary Woods Byrne, PhD, MSN, MPA, RN, is former Associate Professor and Chairperson of Undergraduate Nursing Program, College of Mount Saint Vincent, Riverdale, NY, and current Faculty Associate in Nursing, Columbia University School of Nursing, New York, NY.

Linda Dietrich, MSN, BSN, RN, is Clinical Nurse Specialist, Medical-Surgical Nursing, Bess Kaiser Medical Center, Portland, OR.

Joanne R. Duffy, DNSc, RN, is Assistant Professor, Georgetown University School of Nursing, Washington, DC.

Katie Eriksson, PhD, RN, is Professor, Department of Caring Science, Abo Akademi University, Vasa, Finland.

Kathryn Gardner, MS, RN, C, is Director of Nursing Research/Quality Assurance, Rochester General Hospital, Rochester, NY.

Delores A. Gaut, PhD, RN, is Visiting Professor, University of Portland, Portland, OR, and President of the International Association for Human Caring.

Fredricka Gilje, MN, BSN, is a doctoral candidate, University of Colorado, Denver, CO.

Judith Haber, PhD, RN, is Director, Department of Nursing, and Professor, College of Mount Saint Vincent, Riverdale, NY.

Patricia C. Ira, MSN, RN, is Assistant Professor, Nazareth College, Kalamazoo, MI.

John C. Karl, D. Min., STM, BD, BA, is Executive Director, Samaritan Pastoral Counseling Center, Rochester, NY.

Suzanne Kerouac, MSc, MN, RN, is Associate Professor, Universite de Montreal, Montreal (Quebec), Canada.

Arthur E. Liebert, is President and Chief Executive Officer, Rochester General Hospital, Rochester, NY.

Barbara Krainovich Miller, EdD, RN, is Chairperson, Graduate Nursing Program, and Associate Professor, College of Mount Saint Vincent, Riverdale, NY.

Carol Leppanen Montgomery, PhD, RN, CS, is Assistant Professor, University of Colorado Health Sciences Center, Denver, CO.

Ruth M. Neil, PhD, RN, is Project Director, Denver Nursing Project in Human Caring, and Assistant Professor, University of Colorado School of Nursing, Denver, CO.

Marilyn E. Parker, PhD, RN, is Assistant Professor of Nursing, Florida Atlantic University, Boca Raton, FL.

Lesley Rouillier, MSc, BSc, RN, is Clinical Nursing Coordinator, Hotel-Dieu, Sorrel, Quebec, Canada.

Francelyn Reeder, PhD, RSM, CNM, is Assistant Professor, School of Nursing, University of Colorado Health Science Center, Denver, CO.

Sylvia Rinker, MS, RN, is Assistant Professor of Nursing, Lynchburg College, Lynchburg, VA.

Sister M. Simone Roach, PhD, RN, is Mission Education Coordinator, St. Johns Hospital, Lowell, MA.

Sheila A. Ryan, PhD, RN, FAAN, is Dean, School of Nursing, and Director, Medical Center Nursing, University of Rochester School of Nursing, Rochester, NY.

Carole Schroeder, MS, RN, is Research Director, Denver Nursing Project in Human Caring, and doctoral candidate, University of Colorado School of Nursing, Denver, CO.

Catherine Snelson, MSN, RN, is Instructor, Critical Care Nursing, School of Nursing, Kent State University, Kent, OH.

Beverley J. Taylor, MEd, RN, RM, is Lecturer/Clinician in Nursing, Deakin University, Geelong, Victoria, Australia.

Toni M. Vezeau, PhDc, MS, RN, is a doctoral candidate, University of Colorado, Denver, CO.

Foreword

To the pioneers, leaders, colleagues, friends, and planners, to those of you who dare to suggest, study, and measure "human care as the driving and integrative force for all nursing, and indeed all nurturing of life," it is my privilege and honor to welcome you to Rochester, New York, for what I hope to be your best-ever International Conference on Human Caring.

H. Brownell Wheeler (1990) made the following comments in a recent *New England Journal of Medicine* Letter to the Editor:

> Modern physicians (nurses, CEOs, academicians) are uncertain how to adjust data that suggest a wife's love and support can apparently reduce her husband's risk of angina, even in the presence of severely high risk factors. We tend to dismiss radical cancer cures that appear to be based on faith. We do not know what to make of a study in which survival of patients with metastatic breast cancer is increased three times with self-hypnosis and support groups.
>
> Any new therapeutic drug that triples survival of patients would cause great excitement, great funding, and resultant priority access to care . . . but we simply do not quite know how to handle that "kindness, emotional support, optimism and faith" have quantitative therapeutic activity.

A few months ago we weren't sure we would hold this conference because of the Persian Gulf War. We are indeed grateful that the conflict is ended and that peace may soon be restored. We must, as Mary Ann Bright recently wrote in *Nursing & Health Care*, "expand our focus to include the conditions that perpetuate all wars, factions and conflicts, in the world, in our society, in our communities and organizations and families," which include:

- Unequal distribution of diminishing resources.
- Greed and ego.
- Complacency toward suffering of others beyond our personal circle of relationships (a diminishing community).
- Sentimentalization of "nationalism and patriotism," which in their own right are not wrong unless we use them to rationalize and distance ourselves from the sufferings of others.

As daily witnesses to untold suffering of war victims, soldiers, the homeless, the undernourished, the poor, and the sick, nursing can be an unstoppable force that redirects the fiscal and moral priorities within our country.

Who knows better than you who are attending this conference on care that our vibrancy comes from involvement with others, from contributing our talents and our gifts and our hearts to one another's journey . . . contributing our ears to hear, our eyes to see, our arms to hold, and our hearts to love. When we close ourselves off from each other, we destroy the vital contribution we each need to make and to receive in order to nurture life. Human care is about nurturing life, regardless of its circumstances, conditions or situations.

I invite and welcome you to receive from the many contributions and gifts already prepared for you, I invite you to give to one another for we each need only what the other can give to take back to our communities and families and work places. What a wonderful collection of invitations this community offers. Thank you.

Sheila A. Ryan, PhD, RN, FAAN
Dean, School of Nursing
Director, Medical Center Nursing
University of Rochester
Rochester, NY

Introduction to the Conference

It was a pleasure and a privilege to co-sponsor the thirteenth International/National Caring Conference: "Nursing: The Caring Practice 'Being There.'" In a time when fiscal concerns demand our attention, new technology is a driving force, and the access to and delivery of health care is in question, it is essential that society and health care providers are reminded that our mission is caring for the sick. It is critical that we balance our knowledge of curing, that is, the use of technology and understanding of physiological processes, with our knowledge of humanistic and scientific caring.

The International Association of Human Caring is to be applauded in its mission to encourage and share scholarly and scientific work on caring. This goal places the Association in a leadership role to promote human caring in health care. In adopting this goal, the Association accepts many challenges, including:

1. Preventing the concept of caring from becoming trite. The advertising industry has capitalized on this word. It is in danger of becoming meaningless in our everyday language.
2. Paying attention to the economics of caring. If curing needs to be buffered by caring, how can we afford it, promote it, and enhance it? Research needs to help us better understand the relationship between caring and curing, and identify how this relationship can help to determine how economic resources should be allocated.

3. Helping health care organizations develop a structure and culture where caring is a cardinal characteristic. The interpersonal distance and "red tape" often associated with bureaucratic organizations have been widely recognized as a hindrance to caring. Yet, the complexity of health care requires the existence of formal and intricate organizations. How can these organizations promote and not hinder caring practices of health care professionals?

Nurses have always been advocates for human caring and have served as constant reminders to all health care providers by "being there" with patients. As patient care grows increasingly complex, nurses and other health care providers are challenged to remain staunch allies of human caring in acting as patient advocates.

As advocates of human caring, the International Association of Human Caring leads us to a better understanding of its obligations, complexities, process, and its ultimate value.

Arthur E. Liebert
President and Chief Executive Officer
Rochester General Hospital
Rochester, NY

Preface

The focus of the thirteenth annual caring research conference held in Rochester, New York, was nursing as the caring practice of "being there." The very idea of "being there" can be quite overwhelming, but at the same time we are aware that it is what being fully human demands. Being human is not being perfect; rather, it is a stance of openness to others in respect and dignity. At the conference, the presenters spoke of the caring presence of nursing and patient outcomes; the caring struggles in bureaucratic settings and suggestions for positive outcomes and caring environments; and throughout the conference we have confronted the moral complexities inherent in being present through caring.

This publication includes the majority of papers presented at the 1991 conference, as well as a few invited papers that addressed issues of significant concern. Indeed, this publication has been organized around those areas of concern: presence in practice, caring in bureaucratic settings, caring practice and patient outcomes, the moral complexity of caring, and historical perspectives of caring.

The first group of papers discuss "presence" in practice. In Chapter 1, John C. Karl opens this discussion with "Being There: Who Do You Bring to Practice?" The author helps us examine three essential points—first, the call to practice; second, the difficulty of "being there"; and third, reflections about "being there well." In response to Karl's paper, Sister Simone Roach relates appropriate reflections on practice in her professional career, and

Francelyn Reeder responds as a cosmic sojourner with further insights and reflections.

In Chapter 2, Marilyn Parker presents a creative exploration between the universe of art and the art of nursing in "Exploring the Aesthetic Meaning of Presence in Nursing Practice." She suggests here a paradigm for self-disclosure which facilitates the personal and professional development of the nurse.

In Chapter 3, Carol Leppanen Montgomery suggests that what distinguishes caring as a unique healing communication is a spiritual connection. Through her research, in "The Spiritual Connection: Nurses' Perceptions of the Experience of Caring," the author found that expert nurses know how to care in a way that reinforces their own professional satisfaction and commitment.

In Chapter 4, Fredricka Gilje further explores the interpersonal connection in curing through the universal element of presence. Her paper, "Being There: An Analysis of the Concept of Presence," clarifies the concept of "presence" as a nursing phenomenon and identifies implications for nursing practice, education, research, and theory building.

The second group of papers discuss caring in bureaucratic settings. In Chapter 5, Linda Dietrich studies the extent to which an acute care nursing unit environment was supportive or not supportive of nurse-to-nurse caring. In "The Caring Nursing Environment," the author describes the caring practices, experiences, and meanings of nurse-nurse caring, non-caring, and arrangements and structures in the environment that promoted or inhibited caring within the context of an acute care nursing unit.

In Chapter 6, "Reflections on the Promotion of Caring with Head Nurses," Suzanne Kerouac and Lesley Rouillier describe the process and findings of a participative research study designed to enable a group of head nurses to promote caring in their practice. The caring components of clinical and administrative nursing are explored.

In Chapter 7, Ruth M. Neil and Carole A. Schroeder describe "Evaluation Research within a Human Caring Framework." The authors used focus group methodology to evaluate the programs and services of a nurse-directed outpatient facility serving persons with HIV/AIDS.

The third group of chapters discuss caring practice and patient outcomes. In Chapter 8, Joanne R. Duffy, "The Impact of Nurse Caring on Patient Outcomes," studies the relationships between nurse caring behaviors and the selected outcomes of patient satisfaction, health status, length of stay, and nursing care costs in hospitalized medical and/or surgical patients.

In Chapter 9, Miller, Haber, and Byrne describe a phenomenological study on "The Experience of Caring in the Acute Care Setting: Patient and Nurse Perspectives." The study specifically supports Doris Riemen's pioneering study on the essential structure of caring interactions between nurses and patients and adds to nursing's growing body of literature about the lived experience of a caring nurse-patient interaction.

In Chapter 10, Catherine Snelson proposes a method for explication of the meanings of the domain of trust in the critical care nurse-client relationship. In her paper, "Trust as a Caring Construct with the Critically Ill," she reviews the extant literature and suggests questions the researcher might consider asking the patient to derive the emic meanings of trust.

The fourth group of papers discuss the moral complexities of caring. In Chapter 11, Toni M. Vezeau, "Mothers and Drugs: Two Possibilities for Caring," confronts a clinical situation commonly seen today—a breastfeeding mother who ingests drugs. Utilizing a case scenario to highlight the complexity of such a situation, the author explores two models of caring and demonstrates the differences in the choice of options and in the forms for action for all participants.

In Chapter 12, Beverley J. Taylor, "Caring: Being Manifested as Ordinariness in Nursing," focuses on people interacting in day-to-day encounters. Through a phenomenological lens, she views nursing as humanistic activity wherein the nurse and the patient as humans participate in the ordinary day-to-day experiences of life.

In Chapter 13, Katie Eriksson, "Nursing: The Caring Practice 'Being There,'" offers a different approach. The author suggests that the problem of suffering is connected with the question of good and evil, and that an understanding of suffering is necessary for caring science. The alleviation of human suffering is at all times at the heart of all forms of caring. A caring communion experience requires certain prerequisites, most notably a genuine, mature, and professional attitude. This attitude is something more than neighborliness or friendship, but rather implies responsibility, genuineness, courage, and wisdom.

In Chapter 14, Carole Schroeder expands upon the topic of suffering in a study of some interest, "The Process of Inflicting Pain in Nursing: Caring Relationship or Torture?" The author suggests that while torture is rarely discussed as relevant to nursing, analogies can easily be drawn between common acts in torture and common acts in nursing that inflict pain. The caring relationship resides in the challenge of continual questioning of the beliefs and methods of nursing. In the caring relationship, nurses are compelled to recognize and confront the moral ambiguities inherent in nursing practice.

The fifth and last group of papers offers historical perspectives of caring. In Chapter 15, Sylvia Rinker presents an historical view of nursing as practiced during the American Civil War, "A Caring Presence: Confederate Nursing Practice." The author introduces the reader to the women who dared step outside their "acceptable sphere" to serve as nurses in the Confederacy. The compassionate response of the women to the agonizing conditions of war tells a poignant story of caring in the early years of practice.

In Chapter 16, Kathryn Gardner presents a further picture of conflict between caring and professionalization in "The Historical Conflict between Caring and Professionalization: A Dilemma for Nursing." The author traces the evolution of caring in nursing, discusses the current dilemma related to caring in nursing, and recommends future strategies that will enhance the progression of caring in nursing practice, research, and education.

In Chapter 17, the concluding paper, "The Magic of Caring," Patricia C. Ira suggests a brave new heroine for nurses—The Magician. The Magician symbol incorporates the martyr's emphasis on care and serving others with the warrior's ability to affect the environment by the exercise of discipline, struggle, and will. The author suggests that the mythical Magician construction has a human counterpart in the caring teacher. An historical context is identified and a proposal for research presented.

I extend a special word of appreciation to the officers and board members of the IAHC, INC., the conference coordinators under the direction of Kathryn Gardner and Mary Dombec, the support of

Dean Sheila A. Ryan of the University of Rochester and Arthur E. Liebert, Chief Executive Officer of Rochester General Hospital, and the many volunteers who were vital to the success of the Thirteenth Annual Caring Research Conference.

A very special thank you is extended to the IAHC peer reviewers (listed below) and the National League for Nursing Press editors, Sally Barhydt and Allan Graubard, for this timely publication. It has been the goal of the Association to publish the papers presented at the Caring Research Conferences in a timely and expeditious manner. The energy, and the expertise provided by the authors, reviewers, and editors has once again led to a publication of excellent scholarship in the field of caring. I would also like to thank all of you who purchase this publication. The available proceeds from the sale of this book is returned to the International Association for Human Caring and provides support for the goals of developing and expanding caring knowledge and research.

Delores A. Gaut, PhD, RN
President, IAHC, Inc.

IAHC PEER REVIEWERS:

Agnes Aamodt, PhD, RN, Professor Emerita
University of Arizona College of Nursing
2330 W. Wagonwheels
Tucson, AZ 15745

Anne Boykin, PhD, RN
Dean, College of Nursing
Florida Atlantic University
Boca Raton, FL 33431

Carolyn Brown, PhD, RN
Assistant Professor
Florida Atlantic University
College of Nursing
Boca Raton, FL 33431

Linda Brown, PhD, RN
19007 14th Ave East
Seattle, WA 98112

Nancy Kiernan Case, PhD, RN
Undergraduate Program Director
Regis University College of Nursing
Denver, CO 80221

Kathryn G. Gardner, MSN, RN
Director of Nursing Research
Rochester General Hospital
Rochester, NY 14621

Madeleine Leininger, PhD, RN, FAAN
Professor
Wayne State University College of Nursing
Detroit, MI 48202

Marilyn Anne Ray, PhD, RN
Eminent Scholar
The Christine E. Lynn Endowed Chair in Nursing
Florida Atlantic University
Boca Raton, FL 33431

Francelyn Reeder, RSM, PhD, RN
Assistant Professor
University of Colorado Health Sciences Center
School of Nursing
Denver, CO 80222

Sister M. Simone Roach, PhD, RN
Coordinator Mission Education
St. John's Hospital
One Hospital Drive
Lowell, MA 01853

Gwenn Sherwood, PhD, RN
Assistant Dean for Educational Outreach
University of Texas-Houston
School of Nursing
Houston, TX 77030

Sue A. Thomas, EdD, RN
Professor, Department of Nursing
Sonoma State University
Rohnert Park, CA 94928

Kathleen Valentine, PhD, RN
Director Nursing Education and Research
The Mary Imogene Bassett Hospital
One Atwell Road
Cooperstown, NY 13326

Anna Frances Z. Wenger, PhD, RN
Associate Professor and Director
Nell Hodgson Woodruff School of Nursing
Transcultural and International Nursing Center
Emory University
Atlanta, GA 30322

1

Being There: Who Do You Bring to Practice?

The Reverend John C. Karl

Woody Allen once observed, "Life is just showing up." For those of us, like nurses and counselors, who care for people through the medium of skillful human presence, appropriate questions are: "Who shows up? Who do you bring to practice?"[1] These questions intrigue because I note that, in myself and others, the capacity to be there fluctuates; sometimes we are more there than at other times. Who we bring to practice varies. This study explores these phenomena, but from a perspective which asks this question: "If care for the practitioner's well being were the prime value, what would we find?"

Since I am not a nurse, practitioner will be used in a generic sense.

WHY GO THERE?—THE CALL TO PRACTICE

The Indian myth of Indra's net undergirds my thoughts:

> *At the beginning of the world, the great God Indra tied strands to everything. Earth, sky, clouds, stars, sea, land, mountains, fish,*

animals, birds, plants, trees, men and women, all were connected. The connecting strands formed Indra's net. Therefore, the movement in any one place caused movement in others. Also, the strands were hard to see, almost invisible in some places, invisible in others.

At the intersection of the crossing strands, Indra placed a bell. Thus, one movement effects other movements, and the bells ring. (adapted from Dooling, 1977, p. 4)

Why the bells? The bells sound the connections between things. When these sounds are not heard, connections are forgotten. Strands are neglected, damaged, and destroyed. Holes rip in the net. The web unravels. Life falls through the holes. The bells warn of an ecological justice. As Wendell Berry (1981) says, "You cannot damage what you are dependent upon without damaging yourself" (p. 294).

Who hears the bells? On February 7, 1837, a 17-year-old English girl heard a distant bell toll. She wrote, "God spoke to me and called me to His service." Many years passed before Florence Nightingale knew the full extent of these words. Nineteen years later, the divine voice blended irrevocably with the human cries of the British soldiers who suffered during the Crimean War. Her biographer writes:

But the voices of ten thousand of her children spoke to her from their forgotten graves. In a private note on August, 1856, she wrote, "I stand at the altar of these murdered men, and while I live I will fight their cause." (Woodham-Smith, 1951, p. 181; Dolan, p. 172)

Florence Nightingale heard the bells. She defined a place to stand—the hole in the net that surrounded the British soldiers. She found a way to be there in that place—modern nursing. As practitioner, administrator, teacher, and researcher, she cared for the systemic web of connections that surround the individual sufferer, and thus made visible many damaged and broken strands.

Why go there? The spirit of one's profession defines a place in the net, a particular way to be there, and strands that require care.

Who do we bring to practice? We bring the sound of the bells heard a long time ago, our professional formation, our heroines and heroes, and those strands in the net we care about.

BEING THERE IS DIFFICULT

This paper began six years ago when my Counseling Center, at least superficially, seemed to be improving. The center had reorganized its board, staff, office space, personnel policies, records, billing procedures, and public relations activities. In the middle of a counseling appointment, however, I realized that I had not *heard* the client. I was too tired, burnt-out, and preoccupied to be present. That evening I reflected on a chilling moral dilemma. The frantic pace of "improvements" eroded the capacity for quality presence—the very element we were advertising. The strain of organizational improvements hindered quality service to individual clients. I was caught, therefore, in dilemmas of presence, setting, practice, outcome, and morality. Furthermore, I was not very present at home either. In short, it was difficult being there or anywhere.

The dilemmas resulted in two simple and obvious conclusions:

1. For even the most accomplished senior professional, the capacity to be there fluctuates. One has "good" days and "not so good" days. Being there, basically means a spirited presence, an intunement with the situation and capacity to competently absorb, process, and act. This complex concept involves setting, role, presence, competence, continuum of acceptable performance, and evaluation by participants and community.[2] The point is, the capacity to be there *fluctuates*. Why does it fluctuate? It is limited. One cannot do it all the time. Many situations demand presence—work, family, friendship, householding, self. What happens in one area affects others.

2. The capacity to be there was consistently better under some conditions than others. This conclusion led to a sobering realization. In short, how I ordered my life effected my capacity to be there. I was responsible for who I brought to practice (and who I brought home).

These realizations opened up a new perspective.

BEING THERE WELL—SOME REFLECTIONS

General Perspective

A question frames the total perspective. If care for the practitioner's well being were a prime value that takes precedence over other values, how would that rearrange our perspective on practitioner functioning?

Mayerhoff's (1971) categories are applicable here. When Nightingale cared, she expanded how we comprehend the patient, by enlarging the conceptual "net," so to speak. The patient anchors us in place. The practitioner is committed and devoted to the other's growth. This caring stance reorders values and priorities, and defines strands in the net. But if we really care about the patient, do we not also need to care about what the practitioner requires to be in place, to be there? This perspective enlarges our net of connections. Questions about the practitioner's well being and the conditions that nourish "being there" are now legitimate.

To borrow analogies from Wendell Berry's (1981) work on agriculture, the prevailing industrial perspective only sees value through a lens whose scope is limited and duration short. For example, the value of corn derives from the price per bushel today at the marketplace. Practitioners are viewed as "machines" that tirelessly and efficiently crank out cost-effective service units. Scope is limited, duration short. If we enlarge scope and duration, then the topsoil has enduring value. After all, the topsoil is the source of productivity if not ruined by overuse, erosion, and chemicals (Berry, 1981, 1983, 1987). This perspective expands scope and duration. It places attention on the sources, the topsoils that nourish people's productivity over a consistent, long journey.

This perspective also touches on several issues raised by Sister Roach (1984)—the motivation to care, the influence of settings, and care for many objects.

Important questions are:

1. What conditions enable the practitioner to be there well?
2. What sources nourish, sustain, support, and inspire being there well?

Conceptual Considerations

The perspective forces conceptualizations of the practitioner. The simple question—Who is there?—has interesting possibilities rooted perhaps in childhood "knock-knock" jokes. Every situation involves a "who," an "is," and a "there": abstract notions of individual consciousness (who), environmental shaping (there), and the relationship between them (is). In addition, there are the issues of how we talk about experiences that we commonly label as "inside," "outside," and "between." The work of Martin Buber (1965), Benner (1989, 1990), and Gadow (1990) note similar issues. The problem is to find a language that overlaps inside and outside, individual and environment, who and there, into a *between*. We need a language to blend blue and yellow into green. *Care* is a word of overlap, a "greening" word. It pulls inside and outside into a bond between them.

The following discussion rests on a fundamental assumption: *the more the practitioner is rooted in sources that animate the practitioner's being, the greater the capacity to be there.*

Using a language that acknowledges overlap, we will consider caring about who we bring to practice. Although many categories could be used within this perspective, I will use three: being balanced, being held, and being sustained.

Being Balanced

My capacity to be there was much better under certain conditions of balance, which involved: care of my body, mind, spirit, and relationships. If I strayed too long from tending these balances, presence with clients flattened. I learn this lesson of balance over and over again. When in *balance*, I am more present everywhere.

The concept of balance raises interesting issues. *First*, it implies conceptions of human being; what requires balance—mind, body, spirit, relationships? What are the individual balances of mind, body, spirit, and relationships that nourish consistent presence? We need to note ranges of individual differences. *Second*, balance highlights considerations of temporal duration. What balances are worked out over short durations—hour, day, week? Sabbaticals and vacations require longer durations for professional balance. Are there others that only can be seen through longer time periods of weeks, months, years? *Third*, balance includes issues of value, limits, priorities, and proportion, as well as societal and cultural norms.

If certain balances enhance professional presence, it is important to know what they are; how they can be discussed, studied, and researched; and how they can be taught, supervised, and mentored.

You might think of other questions, but I ask you to play with this perspective: If the practitioner's capacity to be there is a prime resource and value, how do we think about conditions that surround practice and their balances?

Being Held

Mary Cassatt's *Young Mother, Daughter, and Son* illustrates what David Winnicott (1965) called the "holding or facilitating environment." The concept summarizes what happens between mother and child during the first years. "Holding environment" includes holding, feeding, bathing, dressing, touching, protecting, watching, responding, and intunement. The child requires a good enough holding environment to develop emotionally and physically.

Some pictures are worth thousands of words. Look at the Cassatt picture. Notice the mother's holding and the son's being held. Their intunement creates a space between them—the mother's devoted "you're the apple-of-my-eye" look; the child's contented wonderment. Like the daughter, we are pulled into the idealized, loving, being-thereness of the pair. The picture highlights paradigms of care, human bonding, and survival, being there, nursing, the passing of the nurturing art from one generation to the next.

Winnicott (1965) says, "There is never just an infant, never just a mother." As we care about the mothering pair, the picture frame expands and includes the holding environments of marriage, family, subculture, social order, and culture. How the mother is held by this expanding network of environments seriously affects her capacity to provide a holding environment for the child. To paraphrase Wendell

Berry (1983), these are "nested systems within larger nested systems" (p. 46).

There is never just an infant, child, adult, or practitioner. Throughout the life cycle, we live in a series of "holding environments." Robert Kegan (1982) terms them, "cultures of embeddedness" which include the complexities of history, society, culture, and myth. These environments shape and hold us. As adults, we provide holding environments for others. The work of Leininger (1980, 1984) and Tripp-Reimer (1984) illustrate the cultural context of caring practices.

Let us look briefly at practitioner functioning through the concept of the holding environment considering, first, developmental issues, then, work settings.

Developmental. Benner (1984) highlights functional differences from novice to expert practice. Do holding environments change over the professional life cycle? Perhaps the novice and the expert require different types of holding to be at their best. We could study the nature of the holding environments for mature practitioners who are unusually generative and good-spirited. For junior and senior practitioners, those who administrate in educational and health care institutions, those who teach and research, it is important to know the variety of holding that they need and utilize.

Work Settings. Work settings possess great power to enhance or inhibit practitioner functioning. Dysfunctional settings resist improvement and sap morale. Turmoils at work strain other areas of life. In many settings, technological, bureaucratic, and financial pressures can blur and devalue aspects of caring practice. Thus, vital strands in the net are not seen. Caring practices become invisible, or just something extra after the "important" stuff is done. How does one care when the setting devalues it? Settings run a continuum from the oppressive, to dysfunctional, to tolerable, to good, to thriving. Lillian Wald (in Coss, 1989) made this remark about Henry Street Settlement:

> . . . *my definition of love. Someone who brings out the best in you. Henry Street brings out the best in me. (p. 34)*

Play with this perspective. If the practitioner's capacity to be there well were the most valued resource, how would work settings be restructured in better holding environments? Or in Lillian Wald's words—how do we create places that bring out the best in people?

Being Sustained[3]

Our concentration now shifts to the individual's subjective experience of being held. We move from the environment (outer) to internalization (inner), from "there" to "who" from field to topsoil. An example from childhood will anchor this discussion. William Maxwell (1937), in his novel, *They Came Like Swallows*, describes this scene between an 8-year-old boy named Bunny and his mother.

> *Always when he and his mother were alone, the library seemed intimate and familiar. They did not speak or even raise their eyes, except occasionally. Yet around and through what they were doing, each of them was aware of the other's presence. If his mother were not there, if she was upstairs in her room or out in the kitchen explaining to Sophie about lunch, nothing was real to Bunny—or alive.*
>
> *Now sitting in the window seat beside her, Bunny was equally dependent. All the lines and surfaces of the room bent toward his mother, so that when he looked at the pattern of the rug he saw it necessarily in relation to the toe of her shoe. And in a way he was more dependent upon her presence than the leaves or flowers. For it was the nature of his possessions that they could be what they actually were, and also at certain times they could turn into knights and crusaders, or airplanes, or elephants in procession. If his mother went downtown to cut bandages for the Red Cross (so that when he came home from school he was obliged to play by himself) he could never be sure that the transformation would take place. He might push his marbles around the devious and abrupt pattern of the Oriental rug for hours, and they would never be anything but marbles. He put his hand into the bag now and drew out a yellow agate which became King Albert of Belgium. (pp. 14–15)*

The mother's presence, her thereness, makes the child's imaginative transformation possible. When she is there, the marbles become kings and queens. When she is absent, the marbles are just marbles.

Bunny's transformation illustrates what Heinz Kohut (1985) terms a "self-object experience," an experience with another that sustains the self's well being. These experiences developmentally progress from actual experiences with physical caretakers in childhood to a complex surrounding net of experiences in adulthood. For the adult, they include varieties of human relationships, work activities, memories, symbols, the arts, and religion. Well being fluctuates depending upon what happens in this surrounding net. A rich and full net fosters transformations like Bunny's. Kohut believed that the support of the surrounding net is vital for consolidation of the core self, formation of ambitions and ideals, and utilization of individual talents. These experiences often involve subtle and complex senses of another's presence (Wolf, 1988). What are some adult analogues to Bunny's experience?

Kohut (1985), in a paper on "Courage," studied several people who braved death rather than surrender their ideals. Each formed a powerful, idealized relationship with a physically absent "other" on whom they leaned for support as they consolidated ideals. Supported by the sustaining presence, they stood up for their ideals in a barren and intimidating outer environment. In a paper on "Creativity," Kohut again found that the people relied upon the presence of another during times of creative leaps into lonely and uncharted areas.

Who has sat or still sits at the edge of your rug, when you are most functional, imaginative, creative, courageous? Special books reveal new worlds. Conversations with teachers, mentors, and colleagues stimulate our minds. Music evokes memories. Some patients and teachers so impact our hearts that they change the shape of our practice forever. Some dwell in the sustaining presence of a personal God through prayer and worship. In the presence of a few special people, we "reassemble our souls" (Spencer, 1983, p. 197).

Let us think about these ideas for a moment. The caring values of nursing frequently oppose prominent societal values. Kohut's analysis suggests that even when the outer environment is hostile, the self can draw upon empowering internal resources that foster ideals, creativity, and courage.

When being there well becomes a prime value, we need to learn as much as we can about sustaining practitioners. For example, how do we supervise, teach, mentor, and administrate in self-sustaining ways? Because these experiences are so private and personal, yet the very ones that most animate our being, it is important that we reflect upon how they can be shared, researched, and incorporated into our professional lives and settings.

I will offer a modest example. For over 15 years, my counseling center has held a monthly staff meeting that creates a ritualized space in which staff share spiritual resources. Discussed themes are then woven into analysis of clinical practice. The meeting has served to balance professional functioning with spiritual centering, to create a holding environment, and to sustain the self. The meeting allows us to experience colleagues in special ways, to glimpse their souls and what inspires them to be there (Karl & Ashbrook, 1983; Karl, 1990).

CONCLUSION

It is my hope that the practitioner, administrator, teacher, and researcher will be stimulated by the perspective presented here— How do we care for the practitioner's capacity to be there well?

Who do we bring to practice? We bring the sound of the bells we heard a long time ago that called us to professions and to care for certain strands in the net. It is a difficult task. In order to be there for others, we also bring a real need to be rooted in sources that nourish and animate the spirit of our being. And over the long haul of practice, it clearly helps to be balanced, to be held, and to be sustained.

Finally, it strikes me that the conference provides an opportunity to weave a net like Indra's. It provides an opportunity to hear the sounds the connections ring, to see how colleagues care for their strands in the net, and to weave a network of relationships that will balance, hold, and sustain.

NOTES

[1] "Practice" is used in the sense developed by MacIntyre (1984), Bellah (1985), and Benner (1988, 1990). Practices are shared activities that possess an intrinsic goodness. Practices are embedded in communities, attached to history and tradition, involve commitments, and standards of competence. In this sense, nursing, ministry, and farming are practices. The tendency is to abstract out the skill dimension of what professionals do, rather than appreciate how skills are embedded in communities of practice that have history, tradition, and virtues. In this paper, focus is upon a series of considerations that undergird practice and are embedded in the life that surrounds the practitioner.

[2] "Being there" is a very complex concept that involves several elements. (a) There are cultural and social norms and forms that shape the context, assign roles, determine legitimacy, and prescribe normative behavior. (b) For the practitioner, a continuum of subjective evaluation exists which ranges from "getting the job done" to peak experiences "that make it all worth while." A similar continuum of evaluation exists for the recipient. Society and professional guilds also have standards of evaluation. In short, various measures of competency exist. Dombeck (1990) uses some interesting categories to illustrate aspects of the continuum. (c) At higher levels of performance and reception, "being there" is a very complex human behavior that involves maximum therapeutic use of the self. One is present, energetic, in-tune, and has presence. "Flow" is experienced, characterized by deep absorption in the task at hand and performance at optimal levels that couple intuitive and analytical knowledge. Several writers inform my understanding here: Csikszentmihalyi (1990) on "flow"; Deikman (1982) and Ashbrook (1984) on the right and left hemispheric processes of the brain; Schön (1985) on "improvisational" knowledge; Buber (1965) on dialogue; and Benner (1984) on skill acquisition from novice to expert levels. Therefore, "being there" involves setting, role, evaluation, presence, and complex competencies.

[3] "Sustained" is a rich word that possesses multiple meanings and nuances. Its roots are "under" and "hold," thus conveying implications of the underneath—the ground that supports from below. It points to the topsoil, so to speak. "Sustained" means continued duration over time in the sense of to maintain, prolong, keep in existence. It has definitions that highlight the idea of capacity in various ways: supplied with necessities; provided for; to endure, withstand; and to undergo, experience suffering. It has a sense of animating the spirit—to strengthen, buoy up, encourage, comfort. There is an ethical dimension—to uphold or support the validity or justice of. Finally there is a "research," truth-finding aspect as in to confirm,

prove, corroborate. All of these meanings ride along with my usage of the single word "sustain." The support from below, the "ground of being," the topsoil, expands a capacity that can endure over time with an animated spirit that can carry burdens, uphold values, and confirm truths.

REFERENCES

Ashbrook, J. B. (1984). *The human mind and the mind of god.* Landham, MD: University Press of America.

Bellah, R. H., *et al.* (1985). *Habits of the heart.* Berkeley: University of California Press.

Benner, P. (1984). *From novice to expert.* Menlo Park, CA: Addison-Wesley.

Benner, P. (1988). Nursing as a caring profession. (unpublished).

Benner, P., & Wrubel, J. (1989). *The primacy of caring.* Menlo Park, CA: Addison-Wesley.

Benner, P. (1990). The moral dimensions of caring. In J. S. Stevenson & T. Tripp-Reimer (Eds.), *Knowledge about care and caring.* Kansas City: American Academy of Nursing.

Berry, W. (1981). *Recollected essays: 1965–1980.* San Francisco: North Point Press.

Berry, W. (1983). *Standing by words.* San Francisco: North Point Press.

Berry, W. (1987). *Home economics.* San Francisco: North Point Press.

Buber, M. (1965). *Between man and man.* New York: Collier Books.

Coss, C. (Ed.) (1989). *Lillian D. Wald: Progressive activist.* New York: Feminist Press Sourcebook.

Csikszentmihalyi, M. (1990). *Flow: The psychology of optimal experience.* New York, NY: Harper and Row.

Deikman, A. J. (1982). *The observing self: Mysticism and psychotherapy.* Boston: Beacon Press.

Dolan, J. (1985). *Nursing in society: A historical perspective.* Philadelphia: W. B. Saunders.

Dombeck, M. T. (1990). *The contexts of caring: Conscience and consciousness.* (unpublished).

Dooling, D. M. (1977). Focus. *Parabola*, 2(4), 3–4.

Gadow, S. (1990). *Beyond dualism: The Dialectic of caring and knowing.* (unpublished).

Karl, J. C., & Ashbrook, J. B. (1983). Religious resources and pastoral psychotherapy: A model for staff development. *Journal of Supervision and Training in Ministry, 6,* 7–23.

Karl, J. C. (1990). Conversation in many tongues: A model of pastoral conversation. In J. B. Ashbrook (Ed.), *Faith and ministry: In light of the double brain*. Bristol, IN: Wyndham Hall Press.

Kegan, R. (1982). *The evolving self: Problem and process in human development*. Cambridge: Harvard University Press.

Kohut, H. (1985). *Self psychology and the humanities*. New York: W. W. Norton.

Leininger, M. (1980). Caring: A central focus of nursing and health care services. *Nursing and Health Care. 1*, 135–143.

Leininger, M. (Ed.) (1984). *Care: The essence of nursing and health*. Thorofare, NJ: Slack.

MacIntyre, A. (1984). *After virtue*. 2nd Edition. Notre Dame, IN: Notre Dame University Press.

Maxwell, W. (1937). *They came like swallows*. New York: Harper and Brothers.

Mayeroff, M. (1971). *On caring*. New York: Harper and Row.

Morse, J., Solberg, S. M., Neander, W. L., Bottoroff, J. L., & Johnson, J. L. (1990). Concepts of caring and caring as concept. *Advances in Nursing Science, 13*(1), 1–14.

Roach, S. M. (1984). Caring: The human mode of being, implications for nursing. In *Perspectives in Caring, Monograph 1*. University of Toronto.

Spencer, E. (1983). Stories of Elizabeth Spencer. Englewood Cliffs, NJ: Penguin.

Tripp-Reimer, T. (1984). Reconceptualizing the construct of health: Integrating emic and etic perspectives. *Research in Nursing and Health, 7*, 101–109.

Tripp-Reimer, T., Brink, P. J., & Saunders, J. M. (1984). Cultural assessment: Content and process. *Nursing Outlook, 32*(2), 78–82.

Winnicott, D. W. (1965). *The maturational processes and the facilitating environment*. New York: University Press.

Woodham-Smith, C. M. (1951). *Florence Nightingale: 1820–1910*. New York: McGraw-Hill Books.

Wolf, E. S. (1985). *Treating the self: Elements of clinical self psychology*. New York: Guildford Press.

Response to:
Being There: Who Do You Bring to Practice

Sister M. Simone Roach

I want to express gratitude to Dr. Karl for his call to me personally and to each of us here this morning. My way of responding to this call is to relate his reflections to a few rather different experiences in my own professional career.

A number of years ago, I held a privileged position where I found myself to be a supportive presence in a normally tense environment. On a daily basis, I rubbed shoulders with wonderful people in executive-management roles, whose professional lives seemed always wrapped up in the challenge of crisis and change. Not being involved in management/operational activities, I was able to support and sustain and, not by design or plan I might add, I found myself in a position to be that quiet, safe space, nurturing an environment of harmony within a very busy nursing division. There was nothing about this in my role description or in my contract.

As I reflected on this experience in the context of your paper, Dr. Karl, I was struck by the preciousness of such a role as "holder" and "sustainer" for other people, and now realize even more in retrospect what a sacred trust this was and can be for all of us.

My second experience is offered by way of contrast. This was a horrendously difficult situation, where one traumatic change after another compounded an already painful transition for many people. By role and responsibility I was in the middle of it all. As this happened to coincide with the Easter Season, it held all the paradoxes and contradictions of experience in which faith witnessed to joy, peace, celebration, and alleluias; and experiential reality offered nothing but struggle, pain, and a panic for many persons and their families. I kept asking, "Where is Easter in all this?" and reminding myself and others, "while we may not be able to make sense out of this, hopefully, we will eventually find meaning." How did we live that life at that time? Who was sitting at the edge of our rug? Dr. Karl gave several examples of how, in such circumstances, we reassemble our souls. I will try to describe how we tried to maintain ours.

I am privileged to belong to a faith community of women, who by vocation are called to "unity of mind and heart," and to "witness to the world it is possible to live together in love" (Constitutions, Sisters of St. Martha, art. 32). While a religious community shares the weakness and conflicts, the vulnerability and the limitations of any human community, I believe it was this community that held us, sustained us, and provided the "holding environment," the "culture of embeddedness" during this difficult period. This community was the source of struggle and affirmation, suffering and support. We prayed and shared our feelings. One member of the staff who was facing a radical change in her career reminded me of the story of the beautiful tapestry we are weaving but, at times, see only the ragged underside. Even in her struggle, she was supporting the rest of us.

The third example is an experience of being called to be with a group of people involved in a painful ordeal involving one of their colleagues. I did not know the individuals in the group and had only fragmentary information about what had happened. I responded to the invitation with much anxiety and a feeling of helplessness. In a small conference room and over coffee, one by one, individuals expressed their feelings about the situation—disappointment, anger, sadness, helplessness and, in some sense, feelings of being betrayed. While the temptation to intervene with solutions surfaced during this interchange, I managed to resist and listen. My only contribution was to attempt to reflect back what I was hearing from this wonderful, compassionate group of people who were really talking to each other rather than to me. I understand it helped. What they really needed, however, was someone to be present to share their experience and to provide a "safe place" for them to vent their feelings. "Being there" in a particular way was the call of that moment. They needed to "be held."

I am sure everyone here has experienced the fluctuations in "being there" I have briefly described. There is nothing unusual about them. But there is something unusual and unique about our professional role as caregiver which, by its very nature, situates us in the place where all life's dramas are experienced. It is good to be reminded by Dr. Karl that being there is difficult and, if we are to provide holding environments for the people we serve, we need to be held and sustained ourselves.

Reflecting on today's theme, the bells ringing in Taylor Caldwell's (1960) novel, The Listener, provide a fitting conclusion. Her thoughts, paraphrased to apply to the experience of patient and caregiver alike, are relevant to points raised by Dr. Karl.

The most desperate need of people in our society today is not for a new vaccine, or for a specific scientific breakthrough; not for wisdom in interpreting the chaotic, confusing, complex ethical and other issues in the health care world; not for a "new way of life," a new religion, or even for a cure for cancer. We do not need bigger bombs or missiles, the latest in household gadgets, or the most advanced in technological invention. Our basic needs are few and we can survive on a small amount of bread in the meanest shelter. As a human community, we have always done so.

Caldwell observes our real need is for someone to listen to us, not as patient, not as nurse, administrator, physician, housekeeper, janitor, pastoral care worker, but, in her words, "as a human soul." We need to tell someone of what we think, of the bewilderment we encounter, when we try to discover why we were born, how we must live, and where our destiny lies. And our need to tell and be heard is all the more poignant as we experience ourselves as sealed vessels—vessels sealed even to our own thoughts and self-examination.

The "Listener" is that special presence who hears the bells, and one who is capable of naming and responding to the disconnections.

REFERENCES

Caldwell, T. (1960). *The listener*. New York: Doubleday and Co.

Response to: Being There:
Who Do You Bring to Practice?

Francelyn Reeder

    Although there is much to express in response to our keynote speaker, I will be brief. Dr. Karl certainly did more than just "show up" but provided us with a presence that can only be felt through the spoken word after previous thought and careful crafting of the message he wanted to share with us. I want to thank him for the generous gift of himself as well as for the rich fruit of his scholarship.

    Several insights and questions arose during the previous two months as I read his paper and pondered the implications of his message for nursing. My remarks will be limited to three points of special interest.

    First, the Indian myth of Indra's net was a wonderful, inclusive metaphor for an introduction to the paper "Being There: Who Do You Bring to Practice?" The "who" making up the strands within the net included all creatures of the universe, in a dance of movement and response; "Earth, sky, clouds, stars, sea, land, mountains, fish, animals, birds, plants, trees, men and women . . ." (Karl, 1991, p. 1), all called by name. I anticipated the same cosmic thread would be carried throughout the paper. Instead, Karl's story of personal experiences encountered during the establishment phase of the Counseling Center took on more of an anthrocentric focus. One is led to believe that bells at the intersections of Indra's net were sounding and to be heard only between the human strands. I wondered why the expectations associated with being there well did not include listening and responding to environmental realities in and around the Counseling Center? I had thought metaphorically that bells ring and can be heard from many sources if one has a cosmic view of the world. If an anthrocentric point of view is taken, it would mean, in order for Karl to "be there well," that he would have to be directly present to clients, at all times, and in all places. Anything less would be considered neglect and surely not efficacious to sustaining Indra's view of relationships. Such a view also would lead the practitioner to believe that leaving the client to him or herself at times (unraveling the net and leaving a hole) would be shirking one's responsibility to care for other human beings who come for care.

If we looked again at Indra's net and at Karl's situation at the Counseling Center and reconceptualized what are called "holes needing to be mended" or "relationships needing to be sustained," the simple renaming of holes as "spaces" would transform the meaning and expectations entirely. For example, viewed as a "space," one can see in the net a breathing space of hospitality, where all creatures could come and go, or just spend time, by themselves, to refresh and gather the fragments of their lives in the safe, restful, comfort of quiet places of beauty and care. I think that is exactly what Karl was doing, and what many administrators do during the establishment phase of a human service. Instead of being there well face-to-face with clients, personally present, administrators and coordinators need to acknowledge ways they can be there well in practice, broadly defined. As stewards of cosmic resources, tending the space, the initial concern is to hold up clients before their eyes so as to see them in the context of relationships that have woven the fabric of their clients' lives. Holding people's human stories in their minds and hearts during the planning phases of human services requires that the administrator or coordinator assume the cosmic view. Then the creation of compassionate services is possible; for example, creating a safe and healthy environment, setting up sensitive patterns of communication, securing referral and consulting systems, and following through plans that provide just and fair wages for all personnel.

It could be said that the bells did toll for Karl! He did respond! Being there was expressed in his giving attention to developing and creating smooth, aesthetic, and economically sound systems to support life at the Samaritan Center. Being there well cosmologically through space is life-giving for the weary sojourner on the way to compassionate personal caring, because it values the gaps, the spaces between people, solitude, and the road whereon the journey of life proceeds.

I think we can assist each other as cosmic sojourners by sharing our personal attempts to practice the cosmic attitude of being there well. Will we experience fewer instances of "burn out" as we replace our overzealous human respect with an attitude of regard for the larger universe of our lives? This reconceptualization of the context, the net of relationships in life, is critical in nursing practice for being there well.

Karl's attending to these surrounding concerns was an important way of being there well, of being attentive to the environment and of being there in the future for clients for several years to come. Direct service to clients can be misguided unless it is held within the cosmic view, which enhances its capacity "to let go and let God." Whether this is metaphor for some and reality for others, Hildegard of Bingen (in Uhlein, 1983), thirteenth-century mystic, grandmother of creation spirituality, forerunner to Meister Eckhart and Julianne of Norwich, said it well:

> *The marvels of God are not brought forth from one's self. Rather, it is more like a chord, a sound that is played. The tone does not come out of the chord itself, but rather thru the touch of the musician. I am, of course, the lyre and harp of God's kindness. (p. 93)*

I think these words suggest that being there well for others starts with creating a space, a hospitable place where God's kindness, present through all of creation, can then touch persons in marvelous, unsuspecting ways (including moments when we think we aren't even there!).

The second point of my response has already been alluded to in the first one, but elaborates why being there well continues to be difficult. Karl's self-reflections are similar to a historical tendency familiar to us in nursing. Although as a discipline we have widened our transcultural and philosophical perspectives, in practice our usual focus is anthrocentric. That is, primary value is given to persons above all else. However, if our focus remains anthrocentric, then being there well will continue to be difficult because the expectation requires us to give primary presence to persons, for an unlimited period of time. "Burn out" is often the result of a driven life according to the maxim "be all things to all people." We already recognize this phenomenon in our professional lives which easily leads to the belief that "everything depends upon me"; otherwise known as holding a savior complex! Again, a cosmic view deters placing undue importance on our own solitary presence for being there well.

Karl has emphasized the importance of "flow" in and amidst Indra's net of relationships, and has recognized the integral place of the bells at the intersections, sounding between the strands of all relationships. But this "flow" was not carried through the environmental calls of his personal story, the cosmic view again was lost from the analogy. Hildegard of Bingen's creation spirituality again reminds us of a broader cosmic net. The advantages from a broader look at the cosmic net is readily recognizable in nature and in caring situations.

For example, a cosmic view recognizes the ebb and flow of all creation, nature as well as those of human making. We are reminded of the reality that the growth potential of all things, if they are to flourish, needs both darkness and light, solitude and communion, affirmation and negation, giving and receiving; and all these things enjoin the earth, fire, water, and light so integral to the life of all living things. The holes in Indra's net are invitations to possibilities for breath, rest, and to listen, and to be. The spaces between the strands, holes reconceptualized, are clearly invitations to rest. Self-reflecting practitioners of caring realize a special kind of presence, when time is given to discover moments of quiet solitude in the best and worst of conditions. It is a kind of transpersonal presence, expressed by Jean Watson (1985) as "the caring moment" beyond space and time. It is a way of transcending situations for the moment so one can be transformed imaginatively and ontologically on the journey of becoming. In other words, the person whom we take to practice (ourselves) depends upon our recognition of the cosmic view of life. Being one agent in the scheme of things, we too are interdependent and renewed by our openness to participate in the ebb and flow as an equal among all creatures.

The last point of my response is drawn from personal attempts to implement what I call "integrity of self in action" (Reeder, 1991). It is a practice central to the questions Karl asks us to consider when he asks, who do we take to practice! The term "centering" as described by Mary Caroline Richards (1967), in her book, *Pottery, Poetry and The Person*, has been very transformative for me in shifting from a polarity of thought, either/or optional thinking, to a global, inclusive type of thinking. Polarity of thought limits one from seeing the cosmic view and the multiple possibilities and options. It considers only one possibility instead of the multiple options that can be attended to and realized at the same time. The global, inclusive type of thinking, called "both/and" thinking, is more consistent with practicing integrity of self in action which by nature is carried out in the situations of life.

Richards (1973) provides a metaphor I realized was useful for understanding integrity of self in action, as the metaphor depicts processes going on simultaneously in the life of avocado seeds sprouting in a small terrarium on the window sill. Simultaneity is our nature as well!

The metaphor consists of an avocado seed which has sprouted suspended in a glass of water. Long roots, folding around each other, extend to the bottom of the glass (taking in water and nutrients). Out of the top rises a cluster of tiny seedling leaves, green leaves sprouting toward the sunlight, stretching out toward the air for breath (taking in carbon dioxide and giving off oxygen and moisture). The seed rests on toothpicks as it is suspended in place at the top of the water glass. But the wonder of its growth is the simultaneity of multiple and diverse life processes. Living out of an integrated self in the universe is like drinking from an inexhaustible well wherefrom water is continuously drawn (Gutuierrez, 1984); the source never runs dry, but is regenerated in the ecological order of the cosmos! We, like the avocado, participating with the cosmos and all life sources in right relation, are replenished together, equally giving and receiving. The crossing point for us to realize integrity of self in action and a centered presence for being there well in our world might involve living from the heart, being planted firmly in the ground of our being, while responding through a cosmic awareness. In summary, being there well will become less difficult for us, particularly in the practice arena, when we reach a balance of perspective and action. Rather than a goal, balance will be the fruit of a cosmic view of ourselves in the world. "Being held" is experienced and sustained in Indra's net of relationships when we say "yes" to the receiving as well as the doing in our daily lives. The existential bells sounding in the universe of our world call you and me to respond in the time and place where we are planted and sprouting. The cosmic view helps put everything in perspective. An integrated self is then ready to laugh at oneself while taking the whole world seriously (Reeder, 1991). Living from the heart with one's feet firmly on the ground can be very heavy when the lightness and nourishment of the cosmic view is forgotten, for it is only then, in forgetfulness, that we go alone to practice.

REFERENCES

Gutuierrez, G. (1984). *We drink from our own wells.* New York: Orbis Books.

Karl, J. (1991). *Being there: Who do you bring to practice?* Keynote address. 13th Annual International Human Caring Conference, Rochester, NY.

Reeder, F. (1991). The importance of knowing what to care about: A phenomenological inquiry using laughing at oneself as a clue. In P. Chinn, (Ed.). *Anthology on caring.* New York: National League for Nursing Press.

Reeder, F. (1991). *Integrity of self in action.* Unpublished manuscript, Denver, CO: University of Colorado Center for Human Caring.

Richards, M. C. (1967). *Centering: Pottery, poetry and the person.* Middletown, CT: Wesleyan University Press.

Richards, M. C. (1973). *The crossing point.* Middletown, CT: Wesleyan University Press.

Watson, J. (1985). *Nursing: Human science and human care.* Norwalk, CT: Appleton-Century-Crofts.

Uhlein, G. (1983). *Meditations with Hildegard of Bingen.* Santa Fe, NM: Bear & Company.

2

Exploring the Aesthetic Meaning of Presence in Nursing Practice

Marilyn E. Parker

The clay, the pot, the person
The potter, the nurse
All being flows from the center.

Using hermeneutic inquiry to interpret texts provided by nurse artists, the present paper explores this research question: What is the meaning of the practice of art to the practice of nursing of the nurse artist? Aesthetics and presence in nursing practice provide a special emphasis here. To begin this study, however, I would like to share excerpts from my personal journal which lead me to identify and explore the research question.

My experience as a potter has opened new vistas for my experi-
ence as a nurse. It is as if I know truth and beauty in new ways. It
is as if I remember a joining or a unity with all that has formerly
been but is known again after having been long forgotten. Is this
a fresh recall of a universal experience? Is this knowing available

to all who practice certain disciplines such as a form of meditation or yoga? Is this a common and perhaps uncommonly expressed experience of those of us privileged to practice the studio arts? Are there common interpretations of the experience of art in relation to the practice of nursing?

Person and pot are both vessels built from inside with integrity as an acclaimed value of each. Both are living—some say clay dies in the fire, some say it becomes more alive. Is this true also of the person? Fire renders him clear and solid and pure, or he can die from it.

The raising and lowering, the circulation of the clay from the inside out while becoming centered assures that the base will remain whole through the potting process. The shape, the way the pot will be, is determined as soon as the clay is opened and the potter defines the base with movements of the fingers in and out as the wheel moves. Once this definition is accomplished, it is never returned to, is never changed, is only followed. This is the pattern of what is to be, the spirit of the vessel seems to be here. As the clay is lifted, as the pot is made, it is the spirit that makes the pattern that is followed by the potter and this gives form to the creation.

I am nurse, I am with the inner person to respond to calls for help to be what he can be and for assistance to become that which he can become. The person and clay are as one. The clay depends on the person as the person depends on the clay. When I am with the clay, I center, the clay centers. The issues, problems, dreams, longings belong to the vessel, not to the potter or to the nurse.

Some potters say to me "manage the clay, make it do what you want it to do." Some nurses say to me "manage the patient, make him do what you want him to do." I say each vessel knows what it will be and I am privileged to help along the way when called. With both I am creative, am required to ebb and flow, push and pull, center. Both ask for what is wanted and I know ways to sense, hear and respond. Both pottery and nursing nurture me. I am better, more whole, more knowing of myself by knowing both.

SOME PERSPECTIVES ON ESTHETICS AND PRESENCE IN NURSING

All nurses are artists in special and unique ways. The art of nursing is integral throughout descriptions of modern nursing (Frederick & Northam, 1938; Henderson, 1964; Orem, 1991; Paterson & Zderad, 1988; Wiedenbach, 1963). Illustrations of nursing as art have been collected and beautifully presented (Donahue, 1985; Fulton, 1987; Krysl, 1989; Nightingale Songs, 1990, 1991). Art has been used in nursing as a research and practice method and was noted by Nightingale in her concern for a healthy environment (Highley & Ferentz, 1988; Lange, 1990; Nightingale, 1946). Aita (1990) has presented a framework for artistic nursing practice. Aesthetics has been defined and experienced as a pattern of knowing in nursing (Carper, 1975; Schoenhofer, 1989). The practice of nursing of the nurse artist, however, has not been a focus of study reported in the literature.

The context of this research calls for discussion of some views of aesthetics and presence in nursing practice. Aesthetics has historically been defined as "the philosophy of the beautiful," with beauty of an object as the focus (Kinnick, 1979; Runes, 1962). Increasingly, the art itself and artistic processes are becoming the central topic of aesthetics. As a branch of philosophy, aesthetics is concerned with a range of conceptual problems having to do with our understanding of art, creativity, and beauty and goodness in art, including any concepts that we use in thinking and speaking about art (Beardsley, 1966; Kinnick, 1979).

Carper (1975) referred to Munsterberg (1960) when she wrote that "aesthetic appreciation leads to knowledge of concrete experience in its wholeness which is specific rather than general." Such knowledge of concrete experience is independent of any connection other than its own reality. In this context, Paulus Berensohn (in a recent personal communication), cautioned that generalities are false, and stated that the artist is interested in creation rather than in the created; in the power and the process and the healing rather than in the finished object. Berensohn (1972), Richards (1962), and others as well point out that the experiences of the artist can never be adequately described; one can only hope for approximation of understanding. The artist then is concerned with subjective reality, and with valuing the unique individual experience.

Examination of definitions and issues of aesthetics, art, and the artist are essential to the study of the practice of the nurse artist. Presence in nursing practice is recognized as an aspect of the aesthetics of practice and, as a focus of this presentation, will be briefly reviewed. As art, presence, or "being there," in nursing situations cannot be fully described.

Marsden (1990) described presence as commitment in which empathy and protection from dehumanizing effects of technology are hallmarks. Colaizzi (1975) includes mutual openness with the other, entering the world of the other to see the objective from his or her standpoint, and coexisting for some moments in time and space as attributes of presence in nursing. Pettigrew (1988), in her study of nurses' presence with persons experiencing suffering, describes presence as an intersubjective, reciprocal experience characterized by investment of self. This nurse identifies "being there" as a common expression for presence which includes attributes such as risking emotional vulnerability, knowing self and other together, and overcoming distance of separation with a sense of union or joining (Pettigrew, 1988).

THE STUDY

Using hermeneutic inquiry, this study sought to provide understanding about the meaning of the practice of art to the practice of nursing of the nurse artist via interpretation texts provided by five nurse artists.

The Nurse Artists

Each of the participants in the study has experience as a nurse. Three of the nurse artists are studying for an undergraduate or graduate degree in nursing, two are engaged primarily in nursing practice. Each identified herself, or had been identified by a colleague, as a nurse who practices an art such as writing, painting, or playing a musical instrument. All participants have experience with more than one form of aesthetic expression. The study was explained to each one and informed consent was obtained prior to data generation. Each nurse subsequently consented for illustrations of her art to be used in presentations of the study.

Data Generation

Approaches from the intensive journal technique developed by Progoff (1980, 1985) were used to guide each nurse artist in her writing of text to be used in the study. Each was asked to select a quiet place to reflect and write. The nurse was invited to consider first her practice of art and then her practice of nursing in order to more clearly define and deeply reflect on each practice. After reflecting and writing on these two practices, the nurse was asked to reflect and write about the meaning of her practice of art to her practice of nursing. As mentioned, prior to each consideration, the nurse was asked to center herself, to become clear and open to reflection. Topics and some guidance for reflection were provided in writing as follows:

1. Write a few paragraphs about your practice of art. This may be your practice of painting, drawing, potting, writing, or playing a musical instrument. You may consider some of the following perspectives: What is your history with the art, when did it begin, and what have been key experiences in your practice of art? How have your experiences developed over time? What is the meaning of your art to you? How do you feel about your art? What are your hopes and dreams about your practice of art?

2. Write a few paragraphs about your practice of nursing. Again, you may consider some questions: What is your history with the practice of nursing? What are significant times

for you? What is your experience? Key experiences? What is
the meaning of the practice of nursing for you? How do you
feel about your practice of nursing? What are your hopes
and dreams about your practice of nursing?

3. Write in response to this question: What is the meaning of
your practice of art to your practice of nursing?

Analysis of Text

As preparation for approaching the text, I studied hermeneutics
as a system of inquiry in which understanding of a phenomenon
may be achieved through interpretation of text (Allen & Jensen,
1990; Heidegger, 1962; Leonard, 1989; McPherson, 1987; Mueller-
Vollmer, 1989; Palmer, 1969; Reeder, 1988; Wilson & Hutchinson,
1991). I also examined my personal journals which have bearing on
the research question and took opportunity for deep reflection and
writing about my practice of art, my practice of nursing and relations
of the two in my experience. I identified and recorded attributes
which, as researcher, I bring to the study of the research question;
and I identified my needs for assuring optimal conduct and report-
ing of the study. This reflection continued and detailed notes were
kept throughout the process of working with the text. All research
materials, including the approach of the study and the interpretations of the text were reviewed with two colleagues periodically
throughout the study.

The approach to text analysis was done according to my understanding of hermeneutic inquiry. Each nurse provided written pages
of responses to the research considerations, including the research
question. All were read to sense the whole, then the total response
of each nurse was read as a part of the whole, then each part of an
individual response was read as a part of an individual whole. Questions were used to facilitate the interpretation and understanding
by the researcher of the individual texts and of the text as a whole of
the nurse artists.

A description of the process of analysis follows:

1. All of the responses were read in order to obtain a sense of the whole. A statement of initial understanding of the entire text was written.

2. The first part of all responses was then read in order to get a sense of the practice of art of the nurse artist. The first part of each individual response was then read, themes in each were underlined, and all were entered into the computer into what seemed to be categories of responses of the nurse artists to consideration of the practice of art.

3. The whole of the groupings of theme statements was read and reflected upon. Reflection continued as the whole of the first part of each nurse's writing was re-read.

4. The question, "What is the nurse saying to us about her practice of art?" was asked and, as researcher, I reflected on the question and my responses to the question. The results of my reflection were entered into the computer. The question "What is the essence of what the nurse is saying to us about her practice of art?" was then asked, and following reflection, my response was entered into the computer.

5. When all of part one of the entire text had been dealt with in this manner, a statement of my understanding of the practice of art of the nurse artist was written.

6. The process of analysis was repeated for part two of the text in order to obtain a sense of the practice of nursing of the nurse artist. Two questions guided the researcher in interpreting and understanding the text: "What is the nurse saying to us about her practice of nursing?" and "What is the essence of what the nurse is saying to us about her practice of nursing?". When all of part two of the entire text had been dealt with in this manner, a statement of my understanding of the practice of nursing of the nurse artist was written.

7. The process of analysis was repeated for part three of the text in order to get a sense for what the nurse artists had written

in response to the research question. A statement of my understanding of the writing by nurse artists about the meaning of her practice of art to her practice of nursing was then written.

8. To achieve validation, my interpretation of the parts of the text written by each nurse and the statement of my understanding of the total of each part of the text was reviewed with each nurse. Responses of each nurse were noted and entered into the computer. In two instances in which the researcher had questions about expression of interpretation, consultation from individual nurse artists was sought, changes were discussed and agreed upon.

9. Detailed notes were kept throughout the process of working with the text. The approach to working with the text and the interpretation of the text were reviewed with two colleagues periodically.

INTERPRETATION OF TEXT

For purposes of illustrating aspects of the process and outcomes of the method of inquiry, I would like to describe my interpretation of the text of one nurse artist in total. I will then describe my interpretation of the responses of all of the nurse artists to the research considerations about the practices of art and nursing. The last presentation of interpretation is the statement of my understanding of the total text response to the question: What is the meaning of the practice of art to the practice of nursing of the nurse artist?

Interpretation of the Text Written by One Nurse

The Practice of Art. I strive to balance my inner with the outer world; my art lets me know I'm on a path of color and light as healing work. I began using art work in my practice and will probably study those who use symbols as healer or connection to the universal.

The Practice of Nursing.   My greatest ability is as an advocate and comforter. My sensitivity to patients and their circumstances is highly refined and I want to remain open to new ideas and to being present and empathetic to what is missing with the person or environment. I am moved to create aesthetic, natural environments.

The Meaning of the Practice of Art to the Practice of Nursing.   My art and my nursing meet, touch and overlap in being together. A spiral of continuing influence of my art on my nursing and my nursing on my art is created. There are spiritual, transforming elements in my actions. Areas within that are most vulnerable and in need of healing are found. There is connection with what has been missing on some level. I am healed. My patients are healed.

Interpretation of the Text: The Practice of Art of the Nurse Artist

Through my art I am more balanced, healed and whole. I can express my deep personal feelings and emotions safely, creatively and with great personal satisfaction. My art is important, perhaps essential, to who I am. It is a transforming, connecting gift.

Interpretation of the Text: The Practice of Nursing of the Nurse Artist

Nursing is a certain type of caring: to be open, empathetic and genuinely present to help with needs of persons and their environments in sensitive, creative ways. Although it is sometimes difficult, sharing myself with others through nursing brings purpose, meaning and satisfaction to my life.

Interpretation of the Text about the Question.   What is the meaning of the practice of art to the practice of nursing of the nurse artist?

The practice of art is a significant influence in the life and the practice of nursing of the nurse artist. Out of the bringing together of art and nursing new dimensions of caring and nursing are created and both the patient and the nurse are healed.

The practice of art and the practice of nursing touch and overlap in the experiences of the nurse artist. There are many similarities in the two. Both require creativity, dedication and honesty, and both may be responses to leadings but also must be studied and practiced to be known. Yet they remain distinct in ways also; both do not have to be evident together at all times. The practice of art is the more basic practice and preceded the practice of nursing for the nurse artist.

Although the practice of art and the practice of nursing touch and overlap in the experiences of the nurse artist, they are not mixed. While each and both together are dynamic, they are not totally combined into a third entity. They seem to be blended only at the edges where they meet. This form of relating of the practices of art and nursing is evident in the life of the nurse artist and in her practice of both nursing and art. Experiences are new, unique, and fresh. There is beauty, hope, love, freedom, security and satisfaction in both the practice of art and the practice of nursing because of the touching of both in the life of the nurse artist.

The practice of art for the nurse artist leads to wholeness and fulfillment. It is integral to her experience as a person. Art is an avenue for searching and expressing deeply held experiences and feelings. The practice of art is necessary for a sense of full health, and being more fully alive. Through art, the nurse artist feels sensitive to connections with other life and other ways. Through her increasing wholeness she knows qualities of wholeness in others and is quietly aware of the limitless possibilities of each new experience. The nurse artist has practiced several art forms and prefers one or two of them for her own artistic expression.

The practice of nursing of the nurse artist is unique, individual and creative. The nurse artist feels alive and spontaneous, her nursing is loving and caring. Her art makes her a better nurse with her patients and with her colleagues. She knows both the light and dark sides of experience and also knows the nature of the transforming moment. She prays for her patients and for herself. The nurse artist has heightened awareness of relationships, circumstances and environments.

She values, looks for and creates connections of her art and her nursing. She is truly present with her patients and brings forth interactions of art and nursing for the possibilities of healing.

CONCLUSION

This paper has offered an initial exploration of the relations of aesthetics and presence in nursing practice guided by the research question: What is the meaning of the practice of art to the practice of nursing of the nurse artist? This exploration has raised several issues and other responses for further study.

The adaption of Progoff's (1980, 1985) methods of intensive journal writing is worthy of further exploration as a means of generating text for interpretative study. Writing as a group in a workshop format would include opportunity for sharing among nurse artists and could serve to develop depth of exploration for writing individual texts. The quality of environment which could be provided by such a group may also enrich reflective writing.

Some of the questions raised during this study may be considered in future research: What is the place of the study of the arts and practice of the studio arts in nursing practice and education? What are the effects of the practice of art on the being and becoming of the nurse? What is the effect of a specific form of aesthetic expression on the expression of caring in nursing practice? How does the practice of art enhance the fullness of presence in nursing practice? What are relationships between the practice of art and the mutuality of presence in the practice of nursing?

It has been interesting to note the enthusiasm for the ideas of this study and for the reported interpretation of text offered by the nurse artists. Several nurses have identified themselves as nurse artists and have expressed gratitude for the connections made which link the practice of art and the practice of nursing. This has served as another form of validation for the nurse artists who participated in the study and for the understandings described in this chapter. It is hoped that other nurse artists will be identified for participation in other aspects of study of the research question.

REFERENCES

Aita, V. (1990). The art of nursing. *Nurse Educator, 15*(6), 24–28.

Allen, M., & Jensen, L. (1990). Hermeneutical inquiry: meaning and scope. *Western Journal of Nursing Research, 12*(2), 241–253.

Beardsley, M. (1966). *Aesthetics: From classical greece to the present.* New York: Macmillan.

Berensohn, P. (1972). *Finding one's way with clay.* New York: Simon and Schuster.

Carper, B. (1975). *Fundamental patterns of knowing in nursing.* (Doctoral dissertation, Columbia University, Teachers College, University Microfilms No. 76-7772).

Colaizzi, J. (1975). The proper object of nursing science. *International Journal of Nursing Studies, 12,* 197–200.

Donohue, M. (1985). *Nursing: The finest art.* St. Louis: C. V. Mosby.

Fulton, J. (1987). Virginia Henderson: theorist, prophet, poet. *Advances in Nursing Science, 10*(1), 1–9.

Frederick, H. & Northam, E. (1938). *A textbook of nursing practice.* New York: Macmillan.

Heidegger, M. (1962). *Being and time.* New York: Harper & Row.

Henderson, V. (1964). The nature of nursing. *The American Journal of Nursing, 64*(8), 62–68.

Highley, B. & Ferentz, T. (1988). Esthetic inquiry. In B. Sarter (Ed.), *Paths to knowledge.* New York: National League for Nursing.

Kennick, W. (1979). *Art and philosophy.* New York: St. Martin's Press.

Krysl, M. (1989). *Midwife and other poems on caring.* New York: National League for Nursing.

Lange, S. (1990). Using the arts in clinical practice. In M. M. Leininger & J. Watson (Eds.), *The caring imperative in education.* New York: National League for Nursing.

Leonard, V. (1989). A Heideggerian phenomenologic perspective on the concept of the person. *Advances in Nursing Science, 11*(4), 40–55.

Marsden, C. (1990). Real presence. *Heart & Lung, 19*(5), 540–541.

McPherson, P. (1987). The quality of being expressed as doing. *The Australian Journal of Advanced Nursing, 5*(1), 38–42.

Mueller-Vollmer, K. (1989). *The hermeneutics reader.* New York: Continuum Publishing.

Munsterberg, J. (1960). Connection in science and isolation in art, in M. Rader (Ed.), *A modern book of esthetics.* New York: Holt, Rinehart and Winston.

Nightingale, F. (1946). *Notes on nursing.* Philadelphia: Edward Stern and Co.

Nightingale Songs. 1990, 1991, vol 1 (1, 2, 3), P. O. Box 057563, West Palm Beach, FL 33405.

Orem, D. (1991). *Nursing: Concepts of practice.* St. Louis: C. V. Mosby.

Paterson, J. & Zderad, L. (1988). *Humanistic nursing.* New York: National League for Nursing.

Palmer, R. (1969). *Hermeneutics.* Evanston: Northwestern University Press.

Pettigrew, J. (1988). *A phenomenological study of the nurse's presence with persons experiencing suffering.* (Doctoral dissertation, Texas Women's University, University Microfilms No. 88-21422).

Progoff, I. (1985). *The dynamics of hope: Perspectives on process in anxiety and creativity, imagery and dreams.* New York: Dialogue House Library.

Progoff, I. (1980). *The practice of process meditation.* New York: Dialogue House Library.

Reeder, F. (1988). Hermeneutics. In B. Sarter (Ed.), *Paths to knowledge.* New York: National League for Nursing.

Richards, M. (1962). *Centering: In pottery, poetry, and the person.* Middletown, CT: Wesleyan University Press.

Runes, D. (1962). *Dictionary of philosophy.* Totowa, NJ: Littlefield, Adams & Co.

Schoenhofer, S. (1989). Love, beauty, and truth: fundamental nursing values. *Nursing Education, 28*(8), 382–384.

Wiedenbach, E. (1963). The helping art of nursing. *The American Journal of Nursing, 63*(11), 54–57.

Wilson, H., & Hutchinson, S. (1991). Triangulation of qualitative methods: Heideggerian hermeneutics and grounded theory. *Qualitative Health Research, 1*(2), 263–276.

3

The Spiritual Connection: Nurses' Perceptions of the Experience of Caring

Carol Leppanen Montgomery

A s nurses we have lived with this paradox: We are supposed to care deeply about our clients yet our professional socialization warns us not to get "too involved." This socialization "continues to contribute to the devaluation of . . . caring as an affect in nursing" (Morse et al., 1990, p. 6). Recently the over-enthusiastic use of the term *codependency* has reinforced this devaluation by casting suspicion on the motives of anyone who wants to take care of people, which is particularly troubling from a feminist perspective. As Webster (1990) observes, "what used to be the demeanor of a 'good woman'" now falls within the realm of mental illness (p. 61).

Despite this devaluation, as nurses we continue to care and continue to get involved in ways we were warned not to. Certainly, nursing scholars recognize the depth of personal involvement that is necessary in order to care (Gadow, 1980; Peplau, 1952; Watson, 1988). According to Watson, in a professional relationship, the nurse involves herself fully as a person, "including emotional, mental, esthetics, spiritual, and experiential" dimensions of self (p. 66). However, while the literature on caring in nursing supports personal involvement, there is some confusion about the exact nature of this involvement. Aroskar (1991) calls our attention to the "dark and shadowy side of caring" (p. 3). Morse et al. (1990) point out the need for us to address the "unseemly" questions such as can nurses care too much, and can caring reinforce dependency and be untherapeutic. In addition, experience teaches us that inappropriate entanglements in the name of caring do occur. For example, novice practitioners may lose perspective in their overzealous attempts to get involved and rush in and take over for clients. Caregivers may also fall into unhealthy personal entanglements that diminish both themselves and the client. Benner and Wrubel (1989) discuss the narrow path that nurses must walk between *enmeshment* on the one hand and *inappropriate distance* on the other. However, they have observed there is much common wisdom among nurses as to the right kind of involvement.

A research study by this author (Montgomery, 1990) on some of this common wisdom found that not only do expert nurses know how to become deeply involved without succumbing to destructive forms of overinvolvement, but they also know how to care in a way that reinforces their own professional satisfaction and commitment. First, I will describe the research method used in this study, then focus on the core category, spiritual transcendence, a way of being in a relationship that challenges conventional understandings of the helping relationship, and helps to explain how nurses negotiate the complexities of caring.

In this research, I asked two major questions: (1) What is the nature of caring communication and (2) how is caring experienced by the caregiver? I employed grounded theory methodology as described by Glaser and Strauss (1967) within a qualitative naturalistic paradigm as described by Lincoln and Guba (1985). In keeping with the naturalistic view, I assumed that informants were experts with regard to the questions being asked. A pilot study included my own involvement as participant observer during an experience as a psychiatric liaison nurse in a general hospital. Extensive field notes were kept of personal experiences related to caring, observations of nurses, and the content of the hospital environment.

A total of 35 nurses participated in semistructured interviews in which they were asked to talk about experiences that stood out for them in terms of caring, both positive and negative. I recorded methodological and theoretical notes along with the interviews themselves. The initial sampling plan included nurses who were referred by others as representing exemplars of caring, "experts" according to Benners's (1984) framework, with at least five years of experience in their speciality. After saturation occurred with this group, subsequent sampling decisions sought to represent differing dimensions, such as (1) less opportunities for relational involvement (OR, RR), (2) demonstrated noncaring behaviors, (3) felt negatively about caring, and (4) less experienced nurses.

I analyzed data from interview transcripts and theoretical and methodological notes via the constant comparative analysis method (Glaser & Strauss, 1967), comparing and contrasting each individual interview, as well as the different dimensions of caring represented in the sample.

I addressed credibility of findings through prolonged engagement, persistent observation, and triangulation (Lincoln & Guba, 1985). By taking on the role of participant observer during the process of the pilot study I achieved prolonged engagement and persistent observation. I achieved triangulation by interviewing referral sources regarding the reason for the referral, and including this data for analysis. By having all informants review their interview transcripts and by having selected informants review the emerging theory, member checks were structured into the study process.

What emerged from the analysis was an extensive category system that describes caring from a communications perspective, and a model for how the caregiver is impacted by the experience of caring. One theme—nurses assigning a greater meaning to their work—was present throughout the interview data as a concern overriding all descriptive categories and affecting the relationship between categories. I termed this theme *spiritual transcendence,* which I defined from the data as experiencing oneself in relationship as a part of a force greater than oneself. In this paper, then, I will describe spiritual transcendence as central to the concept of caring.

This discussion will be organized around three central features of spiritual transcendence. First, spiritual transcendence defines the unique nature of the caring connection and offers an alternative to empathy as a way to conceptualize this communication process. This allows us to resolve the paradox of how close is too close, and to distinguish caring-centered involvements from inappropriate attempts at helping.

Second, spiritual transcendence serves as the source of energy for caring, and, therefore, is an important resource for the caregiver in managing the stress of nursing. Finally, spiritual transcendence is an integral part of the aesthetic form of caring.

THE NATURE OF THE CARING CONNECTION

Spiritual transcendence defines the nature of the caring connection in a professional caring relationship. Caring, of course, makes possible an intimate form of emotional involvement that challenges the conventional assumption that distance and objectivity are necessary for the nurse to be an effective provider of care.

In regard to the statement above, a post-anesthesia nurse described caring as, "A deeper expression and deeper relationship of yourself with somebody else that you care about. . . . And it's okay to be emotional about it." Informants brought this category out quite clearly during the interviews. Almost all informants became teary or cried openly when recalling significant caring experiences with patients.

Informants also used the term *love* frequently. A rehabilitation nurse described caring as "unconditional love . . . . I think it's hard to stay distant from patients. If you feel for them you are going to enter into their experience whether you want to or not. It's just something that you do." An oncology nurse felt that in order to care she must be willing to "fall in love" with her patients. She described this as a unique form of love that she called "nursing love." In another sense, a medical-surgical nurse described being deeply involved with an AIDS patient: "Even if I was not caring for him I always had contact. I had quite established relationships with his family, his lovers . . . . I didn't know what I was doing until his mother said, 'you know he loves you.'" She described her involvement with him as he was dying: "I helped him hit the pillow and helped him say, 'I am angry.' I was angry too. I have never had that close an experience with a patient who's dying. I was sitting on his bed one day and he was asking my permission to let him go. I said 'I will miss you, [name of patient].'" She experienced his death as a deep personal loss and was still grieving for him at the time of the interview, one year after his death.

However, if we give up the model of detached objectivity and are willing to "fall in love" and become personally involved in this way with clients, how do we maintain our therapeutic perspective, and how do we protect ourselves from the pain?

The literature on *empathy*, the construct generally used to understand the caregiver's role in the helping relationship, would suggest that although some degree of immersion or merger is necessary with the patient, this deep personal involvement is dangerous, and should be balanced with distance and objectivity (Flaskerud et al., 1979; Griffin, 1983; Jordan, 1989; Stiver, 1985).

However, several theorists, including Arnett and Nakagawa (1983), Broome (1985), Gordon (1985), Pike (1990), and Wheeler (1988), in both communication and nursing have pointed to the inadequacies of psychological models to grasp the concept of empathy and suggest the need for a broader framework. To illustrate the limited explanatory power of a traditional view of empathy in regard to the nature of interpersonal knowing, I will share an example of data from the pilot study.

An informant was caring for a man who was extremely anxious about having to face emergency open-heart surgery. He had always lived a healthy and active life, and the seriousness of his cardiac problem was quite a shock to him. He was feeling panic stricken and didn't feel he could go through with the surgery. The nurse tried to calm him down. At one point, he said with great intensity, "I'm just no hero, I just can't go through with this!" This nurse responded by saying forcefully, "Heros are ordinary people faced with extraordinary circumstances, and instead of running away they stand and face whatever the circumstance is!" This hit the man like a "cold wash cloth to the face," and he said, "Where did you hear that?!" The nurse was somewhat embarrassed and told him that she had just made it up. He repeated her statement often and credited her with his getting through the experience. He did well with his surgery and recovery and was allowed to leave the hospital quickly. To this day he visits the cardiac unit at the hospital every year to bring a gift of flowers or candy for the nurses and to make special thanks to the nurse who helped him through the harrowing experience of open-heart surgery.

When questioned about her response, this nurse did not recall ever having felt like this man did, or being in a similar situation which might allow her to identify with him. Her understanding did not involve active projection or putting herself in his position, as empathy is traditionally understood. In fact, her understanding of what she said was not experienced at a conceptual level. She had no idea where her idea came from, at least consciously. Here, then, is a kind of understanding characterized by *receptivity* (Noddings, 1984). The nurse allowed herself to become one with her patient's experience, and, I believe, subliminally received from him what he desperately needed to hear. It was as though her consciousness acted as a conductor to provide the completion of his idea, in the same way an electric current will happen if it has a medium to complete its circuit.

The above example illustrates that caring communication does not occur from a position of interpersonal distance or within a fixed self-boundary. Yet confusion exists as to the appropriate distance and nature of boundaries within which this communication is to occur. This confusion is then reflected in the application of empathy to clinical practice. Flaskerud et al. (1979) attributes the avoidance and distance they found in a study of nurse–patient relationships to the concept of empathy because of its requirements for distance. Even Carper (1978) suggests that empathy be "moderated by psychic distance and detachment" (p. 17). As a result of this understanding of relationships, caregivers are admonished not to get too close and to maintain "appropriate boundaries" (Jordan, 1989; Miller, Stiff, & Ellis, 1988; Pasacreta & Jacobsen, 1989; Stiver, 1985); however, the nature of an appropriate boundary has yet to be specified.

Rather than trying to resolve the paradox of how close is too close, an alternative suggested by this research is to look at the nature of the relationship itself. Analysis of nurses' experiences with caring suggests that there is a distinct qualitative difference between helping relationships connected at the level of the ego and those connected at the level of "something greater." The nurse and the client experience union, but that union occurs beyond the level of self, at the level of a greater force. This greater force can be understood as the "fundamental sacredness and unity of all life" as suggested by Quinn (1989, p. 553), or the recognition of common humanity, shared phenomenological fields, or universal psychic energy all described by Watson (1985, 1988). However, I think that one of my informants expressed this idea most eloquently when she commented that she has the opportunity "to experience a thousand different lifetimes through someone else's eyes."

This form of being involved transcends the usual ego-centered connection, and allows the nurse to become more deeply involved without succumbing to destructive, controlling, and self-centered forms of helping. The focus is never on the self of the nurse. As one informant said, "I was just there." Another informant explained, "I'm not the one, they are the one, and . . . if they are strong, they are healthy, they go on and know that they did that—I didn't do it . . . I appreciate being . . . acknowledged and that . . . but this is their illness experience." Notice that this nurse doesn't try to "own" the patient's experience or make it her experience; she can tell the difference.

Because our culture offers very few models of this way of helping, it is often invisible. In our culture, the predominant model of the hero, the masculine "ego hero," is described by Rushing (1989), as focused on achieving rather than connecting. Therefore, one can see why nurses fail to value or even recognize their own participation in helping others. The goal in caring is to connect rather than to achieve. A psychiatric nurse explained that her earlier immature attempts at caring were characterized by trying to excel, or "get" self-esteem, or prove a point, "jack yourself up," in other words, trying to "have that experience for myself." Now that she has matured, she describes her caring as drawing from what is best in the environment, "going with the flow and being there," or "pulling more out of abundance."

This idea of pulling from abundance implies for me the existence of some greater or spiritual force. Although this spirituality was experienced within a religious context by some, others found their religious assumptions challenged. One nurse described her feeling of spirituality in nursing as

> *a deep sense of ministration to the individual. You minister to the spirit within the body. Sometimes you will not even recognize the person outwardly because of the deterioration. You minister to the spirit. . . . I wasn't aware of that 20 years ago and I think for many nurses it's dormant. Nursing has helped me to discover that.*

For another nurse, "nursing is where God wants me and . . . it's like a commitment of Him, it makes me look at people differently." Another nurse who found her religious beliefs challenged described feeling "more connected to humanity in general." Working with refugees in Thailand inspired one nurse to realize, "people who are in these situations are in a state of grace or in a state of holiness. And so I do think it is a privilege . . . and an honor to be able to be with people like that. . . . As nurses our spirit is what it's all about and we go there." Connecting with a person's spirit, then, allows nurses to find meaning in relating to patients who cannot respond or whose self is hidden behind a mask or physical or mental illness or deterioration.

SPIRITUAL TRANSCENDENCE AS A SOURCE OF ENERGY AND A RESOURCE FOR THE CAREGIVER

Because the energy required for caring originates from a source beyond the self, spiritual transcendence also serves as a resource for the caregiver. As one nurse said:

> *There is an endless amount of love of God for people so I don't even worry about that. . . . I really feel like there is a wealth of love that God has given to the whole, to everybody, and it's available to be used. And so I can love these people with my whole heart.*

The transcendence of the ego also makes it possible to sustain the pain and loss that result from forming attachments and connections with people during tragic circumstances. Nurses are challenged to find meaning when they are "repeatedly confronted with one's own mortality, the inhumanity of others in cases of violence, and the threat of pain and disfigurement" (Benner, 1984, p. 377). As one nurse said, "I feel like in six years I've probably aged 20 or 30 years and I probably have seen more in six years as far as human nature and the basics of human life, more than most people will ever see in a lifetime." This exposure could be experienced as gaining philosophical wisdom, or simply as a wearing down of the spirit. Nurses who were able to grow from this exposure were able to develop a transcendent view of life that would lend itself to a deeper acceptance of what may appear to others as senseless, meaningless tragedy.

Nurses also were confronted with a significant personal experience of loss every time they became close to someone who died. The nurses who were able to cope successfully with this loss had developed a spiritual understanding that allowed for a sense of connection and continuity within the cycle of life and death, and allowed them to transcend the loss. A nurse who changed specialties from obstetrics to oncology explained: "They feel the same in some ways because I almost cry at a birth the same way I cry at a death. It's so poignant at the beginning and at the end . . . it's very alike."

The nurse described above who still grieved for the young man who died of AIDS was able to find fulfillment from the experience in spite of her grief. She described his death as "the most powerful, the most uplifting, the most complete experience. . . . I felt exhausted and depleted, but with a sense of peace and accomplishment. . . . This to me is the greatest thing in nursing. It's the greatest reward."

Her spirituality, which served as a resource for her, developed out of a sense of connection with the holocaust survivors in the Jewish community. She was taught a sense of responsibility to live beyond her own life. This spirituality helped her with this loss because she had a sense of connection with the dead:

I have many images of patients I've lost. They're real for me, they're spirits. . . . they pass life onto me. I am instructed to live

*because they are not able to. . . . I have a responsibility to them
who died so young—to live life fuller, to really be aware of what
life is.*

Another nurse explained how she was able to get beyond the pain:

*As long as you remember people they never die. . . . We some-
times avoid being attached to people in this business because we
are afraid of the pain. . . . and it isn't just pain we should be
looking at. It's the quality of the relationship . . . and sometimes you can't have one without the other. [at this point she
became tearful] And I'm not tearful because I'm sad, that's not it
at all. Sometimes I think tears are a sign of fullness and when you
overflow, you overflow.*

So grief did not leave her empty, it left her so full that she literally
spilled over with feeling.

SPIRITUAL TRANSCENDENCE AS AESTHETIC FORM OF CARING

Finally, the third implication of spiritual transcendence is its
relationship to aesthetic form. Nurses have an appreciation for the
aesthetic nature of caring. As one said, "I pull together a beautiful
symphony." Words such as *orchestrate, harmonious,* and *art form* were
used in describing their experiences with caring. How one knows and
understands the patient involves an aesthetic appreciation. In one
nurse's view, "It's looking at their lives and their gestures and their
behaviors and see[ing] if everything is synchronized."

The rhythm of involvement and standing apart is seen as "an art
you develop as you get older." Walking the lines between burnout and
caring was seen by the nurse respondent as "an art form in itself."

This aesthetic quality lends an enriching or satisfying feeling to
the experience, so that even painful feelings such as grief and
trauma are experienced as patterns of tension/resolution of tension
characteristic of many art forms (Gendron, 1988). These rhythmic

patterns are then experienced on an emotional level as catharsis and fulfillment rather than discord or distress. Thus, this aesthetic quality affects the caregiver's experience with caring, and is another way in which caring can be distinguished from destructive forms of involvement.

The accounts of caring were infused with a sensitivity and response to the subtleties of the situation in a way that was characterized by harmony and grace. For example, an operating room nurse explained how she meets her patients before surgery and extends what appears to be a professional handshake, but by noticing whether they pull back, she can sense at what level they need to be emotionally connected to her. In addition, by reading faces, she tries to get a sense if there is unfinished business between patients and families that may require a little more time before surgery. This reading of and response to subtle nonverbal cues suggests a synchrony and harmony of the nurse with the patient.

The synchrony, rhythm, and harmony that characterizes these accounts of caring also can be found in Gendron's (1988) extensive analysis of caring as aesthetic form. According to Gendron, caring can be understood as total form or gestalt rather than as isolated communication behaviors. I would suggest that this aesthetic form has teleological significance in that it is symbolic of the essential unity of all life.

Several theorists describe an ontologic unity which is distorted by discursive language. Kenneth Burke (1945) describes language as but "crusted distinctions" arising from his concept of reality, which is a "great central moltenness where all is merged" (p. xix). Since language is a selection of reality, it is, therefore, a deflection of reality. Burke's basic ontology rests on the assumption of ambiguity and the dialectic of merger and division. Humans are both separate and unique. We are at once a distinct substance and consubstantial, meaning that we share a common substance. Burke's concept of consubstantiality allows for merger at the level of shared consciousness. By allowing ourselves to enter into this shared consciousness, we transcend the limitations imposed by our own ego boundaries. "We make a kind of ascent from the realm of motion and matter to the realm of essence and spirit" (Burke, 1966, p. 8), where we are all one.

This transcendence can be seen as an artistic process. According to Langer (1957), art takes us beyond the sensual experience of feeling to the recognition of its universal form. For Cassirer (1944), this universal form is teleological in that it "captures a concrete and indivisible unity" as expressed in mythic consciousness where thought is not "divided into classes and subclasses. . . . It is felt as an unbroken continuous whole" (p. 81).

Art according to Burke (1966) is "the creation of an appetite in the mind of the auditor, and the adequate satisfying of that appetite" (p. 31). During the artistic moment of caring, the appetite is for what is promised by the relationship: a connection. And if caring succeeds, this connection is one that transcends self, time, and space, and allows access to a primary universal energy in the manner described by Watson (1988). This then transcends the separation between the nurse and the client and frees both from their separation and loneliness (Watson, 1988).

In summary, what distinguishes caring as a unique healing communication is that its connection is beyond the level of ego, at the level of spirit. This transcendence of ego allows caregivers to become deeply involved without succumbing to destructive forms of overinvolvement. The spiritual nature of the connection also serves as an important resource from which the caregiver can derive meanings that sustain him or her through loss and other stressors associated with caring. Finally, spiritual transcendence artistically represents a greater unity, releasing us from our isolation. While caring (and the results of this research are far more complex than this paper can capture), I offer this central theme of spiritual transcendence as a centering point. If caring is the essence of nursing (Leininger, 1978), then transcending one's ego to find a greater meaning in the relationship may be the essence of caring.

REFERENCES

Arnett, R. C., & Nakagawa, G. (1983). The assumptive roots of empathic listening: A critique. *Communication Education*, (32), 368–378.

Aroskar, M. A. (1991). Caring—Another side. *Journal of Professional Nursing*, 7(1), 3.

Benner, P. (1984). *From novice to expert: Excellence and power in clinical nursing practice.* Menlo Park, CA: Addison Wesley.

Benner, P., & Wrubel, J. (1989). *The primacy of caring.* Menlo Park, CA: Addison Wesley.

Broome, B. J. (1985). *A reconceptualization of empathy and its role in interpersonal communication.* (report No. CS 505 161) Fairfax, VA: George Mason University. (Eric Document Reproduction Service No. ED 265 584).

Burke, K. (1945). *A grammar of motives.* Berkeley: University of California Press.

Burke, K. (1950). *A rhetoric of motives.* Berkeley: University of California Press.

Burke, K. (1966). *Language as symbolic action: Essays on life, literature, and method.* Berkeley: University of California Press.

Carper, B. A. (1978). Fundamental patterns of knowing in nursing. *Advances in Nursing Science, 1*(1), 12–23.

Cassirer, E. (1944). *Essay on man.* Fredricksberg, VA: Yale University Press.

Flaskerud, J. H., Halloran, E. J., Janken, J., Lund, M., & Zetterlund, J. (1979). Avoidance and distancing: A descriptive view of nursing. *Nursing Forum, 18*(2), 158–175.

Gadow, S. (1980). Existential advocacy: Philosophical foundation of nursing. In S. Spicker & G. Gadow (Eds.), *Nursing images and Ideals.* New York: Springer, 86–101.

Gendron, D. (1988). The expressive form of caring. *Perspectives in caring monograph 2.* Toronto: University of Toronto.

Glaser, B. G., & Strauss, A. L. (1967). *The discovery of grounded theory: Strategies for qualitative research.* New York: Adeline.

Gordon, R. D. (1985, August). *The search for multimethodological approaches to empathic communication development* (Report No. CS 505 011) Honollulu, Hawaii: University of Hawaii. (Eric document Reproduction Service No. ED 261 419).

Griffin, A. P. (1983). A philosophical analysis of caring in nursing. *Journal of Advanced Nursing, 8,* 289–295.

Jordan, J. (1989). *Relational development: Therapeutic implications of empathy and shame.* Stone Center tapes. (Available from Stone Center, Wellesley College, Wellesley, MA).

Langer, S. K. (1957). *Philosophy in a new key.* Cambridge: Harvard University Press.

Leininger, M. (1978). The phenomenon of caring. Part V. *Nursing Research Report, 12*(1), 2–14.

Lincoln, Y. S., & Guba, E. G. (1985). *Naturalistic inquiry.* Newbury Park: Sage.

Miller, K. I., Stiff, J. B., & Ellis, B. H. (1988). Communication and empathy as precursors to burnout among human service workers. *Communication Monographs, 55*, 250–265.

Montgomery, C. L. (1990). Nurses' perceptions of significant caring communication encounters. *Dissertation Abstracts International, 51-07A*, 2198. (University Microfilms No. AAD 90-30091).

Morse, J. M., Solberg, S. M., Neander, W. L., Bottorff, J. L., & Johnson, J. L. (1990). Concepts of caring and caring as a concept. *Advances in Nursing Science, 13*(1), 1–14.

Noddings, N. (1984). *Caring: A feminine approach to ethics and moral development.* Berkeley: University of California Press.

Pasacreta, J. V., & Jacobson, P. B. (1989). Addressing the need for staff support among nurses caring for the AIDS population. *Oncology Nursing Forum, 16*(5), 658–662.

Peplau, H. E. (1952). *Interpersonal relations in nursing.* New York: Putnam.

Pike, A. W. (1990). On the nature and place of empathy in clinical nursing practice. *Journal of Professional Nursing, 6*(4), 235–241.

Quinn, J. F. (1989). On healing, wholeness, and the haelan effect. *Nursing and Health Care, 10*(10), 553–556.

Rushing, J. H. (1989). Evolution of "the new frontier" in Alien and Aliens: Patriarchal co-optation of the feminine archetype. *The Quarterly Journal of Speech, 75*(1), 1–24.

Stiver, I. F. (1985). The meaning of care: Reframing treatment models. *Work in progress series: Stone Center for developmental services and studies.* Wellesley MA.: Wellesley College.

Watson, J. (1985). *Nursing: Human science and human care.* Norwalk, CT: Appleton Century Crofts.

Watson, J. (1988). *Nursing: Human science and human care: A theory of nursing.* New York: National League for Nursing.

Webster, D. (1990). Women and depression (alias codependency). *Family and Community Health, 13*(3), 58–66.

Wheeler, K. (1988). A nursing science approach to understanding empathy. *Archives of Psychiatric Nursing, 2*(2), 95–102.

4

Being There: An Analysis of the Concept of Presence

Fredricka Gilje

Presence is a universal element of interpersonal phenomenon. For nurses, the importance of presence has been known intuitively for some time. Now, however, this elusive interpersonal, intrapersonal, and transpersonal phenomenon is beginning to be recognized and articulated as a valuable dimension of human experience.

Because the concept of presence has yet to be fully defined or described in nursing, concept analysis and development have become priorities. Here, concept analysis becomes a necessary process for clarifying ways of knowing about phenomena and developing a knowledge base for nursing.

In this paper, then, I will focus on an analysis of the concept of presence, using process strategies described by Wilson (1969) and related to nursing theory by Chinn and Jacobs (1991), and Walker and Avant (1983). There is a twofold purpose here: (1) to clarify the concept of presence as a nursing phenomenon and (2) to begin to identify implications this concept has for nursing practice, education, research, and theory building.

LITERATURE REVIEW

The work of Patterson and Zderad (1988), two psychiatric mental health nursing theorists published in the 1970s, stimulated awareness of *presence* as a powerful phenomenon in nursing. During the 1980s, published research on the concept of caring proliferated and heightened awareness of presence as a component of the caring process. In this regard, presence has been implicitly or explicitly identified in numerous nursing theories such as Watson's human caring (1985), Parse's man-living-health theory (1981), Roger's science of unitary human beings, and Patterson and Zderad's humanistic nursing.

A review of nursing literature on presence and presencing since 1980 revealed limited publications on the topic. Two nursing authors used the concept of presence and presencing for chapter titles in books, one of which concerns nursing interventions (Gardner, 1985) while the other concerns nursing research (Wilson, 1986). In my awareness, these are the two nursing sources which have, to any extent, described and somewhat analyzed presence as a concept. Otherwise, several published research articles on caring have identified presence as a component of caring (Cronin & Harrison, 1988; Forest, 1989; Hinds, Martin, & Vogel, 1987; Larson, 1987; Mayer, 1986; Swanson-Kauffman, 1986).

In my examination of the concept of presence, and for the purpose of this paper, I will focus on a phenomenological-existential-humanistic view of person. This philosophical basis clarifies the value of person and constructs a reality that encompasses *being* as an integral component of meaningful interpersonal experiences via descriptions of being by Heidegger (1987) and Buber (1965). In nursing particularly, authors such as Benner and Wrubel (1989), Fawcett (1984), Hudson (1988), Leininger (1986), and Leonard (1989) have addressed person as a central concept.

In reviewing nursing literature, then, it is evident that an ontological perspective needs to be valued and explored. According to Leonard (1989), in fact, nursing needs to focus on what it means to be a human being.

A LINGUISTIC EXAMINATION

According to dictionary sources, the word *presence* is used as a noun, a synonym, and the object of a verb (Grove, 1963, p. 1973; Oxford English Dictionary, 1961, p. 1300). Definitions and uses of the word *presence* reveal several common perceptions. Seven definitions are identified and illustrated for the purpose of gaining a clearer understanding of the concept.

Presence *as* Being

A common recurring definition and use of the word *presence* is *being*. *Being* as a noun is commonly defined as "existence" and "actuality" (Merriam-Webster, 1988). A synonym for *being* is *essence*. Essence can be defined as "the most basic, significant and indispensable element, attribute, quality, property or aspect of a thing" (Merriam-Webster, 1988). In dealing with the philosophical basis for *being*, both Heidegger (1987) and Buber (1965) offered powerful descriptions. According to Heideggerian phenomenology, the fundamental question is "What is it like to be a person?" Heidegger strongly asserted that *being* is the essence or core of a person. According to Buber, *being* is dependent upon the relationship between the "I" and the "thou." For Buber, reality is "being-in-between" which is characterized by mutuality and presentness. The "I-Thou" focuses on the whole *being* and begins from experience. *Being* then is the very personal, individual, unique attribute, quality, or spirit which makes one human. As described by Heidegger, *being* can be experienced by sharing one's *presence*. As described by Buber, *being* also can be experienced by being in relationship to and with others.

Presence *as* Being Here *and* Not Elsewhere

A very simple but succinct definition of the word *presence* is a "state of being in one place and not elsewhere" (Grove, 1963, p.

1793). In this perspective, presence is "existing in a single situation, position, location, or portion of space" (Merriam-Webster, 1988, p. 556). "Here" is an antonym to "elsewhere" implying a difference in place.

This definition can be interpreted as having a psychological or a physical component. From a concrete viewpoint, environments or geographic locations which have personal meaning, such as home, school, or church, can be considered as places of existence or *being*. An illustration, then, of *being here* and *not elsewhere* is: A woman visited her childhood home where relatives or family members no longer resided. In that environment, she was physically located in a place which evoked memories of her parents, siblings, and friends who had been so much a part of her childhood years.

Presence *as* Being There *and* Being With

A common dictionary definition of *presence* is "closeness" which means nearness in time, space, amount, or resemblance (Oxford University Dictionary, 1961, p. 519). Individuals experience closeness not only physically but also in a psychological, emotional, and spiritual realm.

Patterson and Zderad (1988), in defining and delineating the concept of *presence*, explicitly identified two components: the physical and the psychological. Gardner (1985) reiterated Patterson and Zderad's definition of *presence* in terms of nursing as the physical "being there" and the psychological "being with" a patient.

Although the physical component of *presence* is quite concrete and easily grasped—as characterized by a temporal-spatial relationship—the psychological component is more abstract and difficult to describe and articulate.

As described by Gardner (1985), the psychological component refers to an intuitive knowing whereby the nurse senses the patient's experience. This significant dimension of *presence* was more clearly explicated by Newman (1986) and Watson (1985). For

Newman, the psychological component of *presence* can be understood in a relational paradigm that encompasses consciousness and is characterized by a pattern of person-environment-interaction which is acausal, intuitive, and probabilistic.

For Watson (1985), the psychological component of *presence* includes the psychological, social, emotional, ethical, and spiritual realms which directly impact the caring process. Watson described the art of nursing as a human activity which involves a union of feelings. For Watson, this unity of feelings encompasses a transmission of the soul through full use of self. Conditions of this process include the nurse's use of spirituality, individuality, and sincerity.

Being there and *being with* are revealed in the following example: A nurse calmly approached and acknowledged a patient with his preferred name in an authentic way. She situated herself comfortably in a chair, conscious of her thoughts, feelings, and actions. The patient and nurse mutually shared self disclosure. The nurse reflected on and affirmed the patient's deep feelings considering the context of his experience. The patient sensed the nurse's compassion and felt understood.

Another example of *being there* and *being with* in a psychological sense is illustrated in anniversary reactions. In these instances, an individual relives the presence of significant events experienced at a previous time and date. Anniversary reactions may occur on anniversaries of deaths, divorces, weddings, and so on.

A related case example of *being there* but not *being with* is stated as follows: A nurse entered a patient's room and immediately checked the interveneous equipment without making eye contact with or verbally acknowledging the patient; she was not conscious of the patient's needs or desires. After checking the IV, she briskly left the room.

As technical skills in health care have advanced, our appreciation for human identity and esteem, that is, human being, are at risk. Unfortunately, in many settings, health care professionals have focused more on procedures and methods than on *being there* and *being with*.

Presence *as* Existence *or* Influence

The word *presence* also is defined as "one having existence or influence in the present" (Grove, 1963, p. 1793; Oxford Unabridged Dictionary, 1961, p. 1300). The focus of this definition falls on the words *existence* and *influence*. A synonym for *existence* is *being* or *actuality* (Merriam-Webster, 1988, p. 285). *Influence* can be defined as "power exerted over the minds or behavior of others" (Merriam-Webster, 1988, p. 407). According to Patterson and Zderad (1988), this view of *presence* incorporates a transforming quality that results in change.

Wilson (1986) included the influencing act of intervention as one stage in her concept of *presencing*. According to Wilson, intervention included active and passive strategies intended to "control" situations. Examples focusing on *existence* as *being* have been given in previous sections of this paper. The following scenario provides a more specific example of *presence* as having influence: A nurse administrator was known for her respect of others and facilitation of an atmosphere of mutuality and equalitarianism. She welcomed ideas, sought options, and advocated participatory management. When she wasn't physically present, her expectations permeated the environment and effected attitudes and decisions of the staff.

Presence *as* Feeling *or* Believing

Another definition of *presence* is "something felt or believed to be present" (Grove, 2963, p. 1793; Oxford Unabridged Dictionary, 1961, p. 1300). According to Quinn (1988), in this perspective of *presence*, a person's significant relationships with inanimate objects which have symbolic meaning as well as having spiritual beliefs and experiences tied to them can be described. Considerations of transcendental experiences may be useful in actualizing this definition: For some individuals, going into a church or synagogue evokes a meaningful feeling of awe and a belief in the *presence* of a higher being. Other examples of *presence* as "something felt or believed" are found in prayer, religious symbols, pictures, or objects which evoke feelings of significance for the individual.

In addition to positive effects or outcomes of presence, negative or undesirable consequences occur when *presence* is inappropriately used. An undesirable outcome or contrary case is apparent in the following example: A newly admitted psychiatric patient was approached by the nurse. The nurse introduced herself. The patient replied in a hostile voice, "You are making me nervous. I don't want to talk to anyone now. I just want to be alone." The nurse acknowledged the patient's response, said she would be available to talk later, and walked away.

Here, the nurse recognized the patient's expressed temporal spatial needs and appropriately removed herself from the patient.

Presence *as* Caring

In recent literature and research, *presence* has been associated with caring. In a phenomenological study conducted by Riemen in 1986, the researcher analyzed patients' descriptions of noncaring nurse–patient interactions. In this study, noncaring was evidenced by nonpresence and distance of the nurse.

In another phenomenological study, Forest (1989) investigated caring from nurses' perceptions. Here, a priority theme *being there* evolved. Results indicated that the essential structure of caring "is first and foremost a mental and emotional presence that evolves from deep feelings for the patient's experience" (p. 818).

In another study, Brown (1986) identified *presence* as one of eight themes of care as perceived by hospitalized patients. "Although the nurse did various things in the interaction, the quality that was most important to the patient's experience of care was the reassuring presence of the nurse" (p. 59).

Hinds, Martin, and Vogel (1986) explored hopefulness in adolescent oncology patients. A key finding identified that adolescents perceived the "nurse's personal commitment" and involvement as a meaningful strategy. In this study, reported data inferred the value of the *presence* of the nurse. Findings in three separate studies by Cronin and Harrison (1988), Larson (1987) and Mayer (1986) revealed similar perceptions of nurse caring behaviors as reported by patients with an oncological problem or myocardial infarction.

Absence of Presence

A concept can frequently be better understood by examining its opposite. An antonym for *presence* is *absence*. One's *presence* can be absent not only in the physical realm but also in the psychological, emotional, and spiritual realms. Absence of presence has been illuminated as absence of relationship (Buber, 1970; Marcel, 1965; Riemen, 1986; Scarry, 1985) and absence of the soul (Daly, 1984).

Absence of *presence* as absence of relationship is manifest in a myriad of social and emotional problems such as substance abuse, violence, and some mental illnesses. In Riemen's (1986) findings, noncaring as nonpresence was degrading, belittling, and expressed a lack of concern. In highly technological procedures, objectification of patients results in absence of relationship.

Mary Daly (1984) has discussed an ontological perspective of *presence* from a feminist and existential view. Daly described absence of *presence* here as "absence of the soul." Such an absence occurs in myths, ideologies, and traditions which are perpetuated from generation to generation and which stifle creativity and growth, resulting in meaninglessness. According to Daly, for example, it is through oppressive practices, perpetuated by patriarchial myths, ideologies, and traditions, that women become bound to roles in an existence that they suffer. In addition, women who have assumed a multitude of invisible roles that contribute to society, remain in one form or another absent from the *presence* of patriarchal institutional values. Daly strongly advocated that absence of *presence* be cast off and replaced with a new meaningful reality of being ontologically valued in society. These realities directly affect nursing and challenge the profession to test new ways of knowing and doing which are purposive and meaningful.

DELINEATION OF "PRESENCE"

In each of the definitions and descriptions of *presence*, common critical attributes as well as antecedent and outcome criteria were apparent. The major defining attribute of *presence* was the ability to psychologically or emotionally *be with* or *attend to* a person, place, or object. The major antecedent of *presence* was a temporal spatial connection with a person, place, or object.

According to the current literature, *being with* was the most consistently used definition of the word *presence*. A proposed theoretical definition for nursing of the concept *presence* is "an intersubjective and intrasubjective energy exchange with a person, place, object, thought, feeling, or belief that transforms sensory stimuli, imagination, memory, or intuition into a perceived meaningful experience." This definition embodies and requires congruence of body, mind, and spirit. Integral to this definition is the inclusion of a reflective state of consciousness as a key element. In this regard, valuing *being* and knowing are essential processes for understanding the concept and applying it to human experiences.

The outcomes which unfold and evolve subsequent to *presence* are numerous, indicating the many benefits that *presence* can have in interpersonal experiences. These outcomes, referred to as consequences by Walker and Avant (1983), include social, spiritual, psychological, and physical dimensions for the patient as well as the nurse.

Outcomes of *presence* have an affirming or disconfirming effect on interpersonal and intrapersonal experiences. An experience with *presence* may result in an experience of love (Liehr, 1989); meaning and purpose (Quinn, 1984); hope (Hinds, Martin, & Vogel, 1987; Patterson & Zderad, 1988); transpersonal caring (Watson, 1988); self-disclosure (Johnson, 1980); and expansion of consciousness (Newman, 1986). On the other hand, depending upon individual needs and perceptions, *presence* also can result in loneliness, alienation, isolation (Quinn, 1988), disengagement, and increased anxiety.

Subsequent advantages of the use of *presence* in nursing include lingering presence (Benner & Wrubel, 1989); intuitive knowledge (Chinn & Jacobs, 1991); advocacy (Gadow, 1979; Gadow, 1980); and healing (Quinn, 1988). As further knowledge of mind–body interaction is valued and more completely understood, the possible outcomes of the nurse's *presence* could expand.

Analysis of *presence* revealed concepts from which *presence* must be delineated. In this regard, delineating concepts similar to or different from the concept undergoing analysis clarified the meaning and understanding of the term.

Empathy is a concept somewhat related to *presence*. Upon initial consideration, *presence* may seem very similar to *empathy*. However, closer scrutiny reveals the concepts as having differing attributes as well as antecedents and outcomes.

According to Travelbee (1971), *empathy* is defined as a "process wherein an individual is able to see beyond outward behavior and sense accurately another's inner experience at a given point in time" (p. 136). Antecedents to empathy, as described by Travelbee, include: similarities of experiences between the people involved and the desire to comprehend or understand another which may be motivated by curiosity (p. 138). Travelbee further described empathy as a one-way process which may or may not result in constructive growth. She stated that "emotional and intellectual knowledge may be used to help the other person, or it may be used to manipulate and exploit the other person" (p. 139).

Empathy, then, according to Travelbee, involves an objective perspective in which cognitive and predictive attributes are paramount and awareness and experiencing of the others' reactions, feelings, and concerns may not necessarily occur. In addition, Travelbee saw "similarities of experience" as a prerequisite to empathy. This prerequisite is quite contrary to the emphasis described in more recent caring literature in which *presence* can be viewed as *being with* and sharing feelings of another in a mutual and reciprocal manner.

Outcomes of empathy as delineated by Travelbee included: comprehending meaning and relevance of thoughts and feelings of the individual concerned; closeness; mutual concern; predicting another's behavior; meaning; rapport; value judgments; and exploitation. Except for exploitation and predicting, of course, these outcomes are the same as for *presence*.

It is quite apparent that *presence* and *empathy* are based on differing philosophical thoughts. Whereas *presence* has its basis in Heidegger and Buber as earlier described, *empathy*, as described by

Travelbee, is based on positivistic influence which is evident in the dualistic, separate, and uninvolved role of the nurse as a person. In this focus, the nurse, for example, relates to the other as an object in an effort to consciously predict the other's behavior. Although empathy has been used and developed by various professions since the early 1970s, perhaps it is outdated and a new way is needed to begin to articulate the complexity of interpersonal processes within a caring context.

In contrast, *presence* is part of a holistic caring approach which involves integration of mind, body, and spirit. This somewhat invisible and indivisible process results in transpersonal caring as described by Watson (1985). Such caring is transforming and has the potential to alter experiences for the patient as well as the nurse. Instead of cognitive forces only occurring between those with similar experiences, *presence* can occur in the absence of similar experiences and based solely on an appreciation of and for humanity. The sharing of humanness comes from the inside out and can transcend our likes and dislikes for anther person.

NURSING IMPLICATIONS

Understanding the concept of *presence* has several significant implications for nursing education, nursing practice, and nursing research. The primary implication is philosophical. Valuing ontology creates philosophies of nursing which are not merely formal linguistic exercises, but instead are meaningful beliefs reflected in practice. For nursing, this requires addressing *person* as a central concept as indicated by Benner and Wrubel (1989), Fawcett (1984), Hudson (1988), Leininger (1986), and Leonard (1989).

Here valuing *person* embraces the contextual aspect of existence which occurs in relationship with others. Through *presence*, persons experience ethical, aesthetic, empirical, and personal ways of knowing as described by Carper (1985) as well as Chinn and Jacobs (1987). Only through valuing *presence* can the nurse be concerned not only with "well being" but with "more being" and "becoming" as described by Patterson and Zderad (1988, p. 12).

For an extensive period of time, nursing practice, education, and research have promoted and actually reinforced a concrete, tangible reality based on a medical model of objectism and reductionism with emphasis on technology, procedures, and content. This emphasis has far outweighed the importance of a patient as a human being, of a student as a human being, of a nurse as a human being, or of a research participant as a human being.

In this form of concept analysis, nurses can reach a clearer communication and understanding of *presence,* a key element in their interactions with clients as well as professional staff. In addition, this information may stimulate a reassessment of the value of the nurse's *presence* which is, or should be, central to the profession of nursing.

CONCLUSION

There is in nursing literature a beginning awareness of the significance of the concept *presence.* As a key concept in interpersonal, intrapersonal, and transpersonal phenomena, *presence* is certainly a concern to nursing. While nurses have frequently shared *being with* patients in many meaningful ways, although usually at an unconscious level of awareness, today we must challenge ourselves to create ways of knowing and valuing this information.

In this paper, I have attempted to define, describe and delineate the concept of *presence.* Still, however, more research is needed to reveal the value of *presence* as an intricate, forceful concept in nursing.

REFERENCES

Benner, P., & Wrubel, J. (1989). The primacy of caring. Menlo Park, CA: Addison Wesley.

Brown, L. (1986). The experience of care: Patient perspectives. *Topics in Clinical Nursing, 8*(2), 56–62.

Buber, M. (1965). The knowledge of man. New York: Harper and Row.

Carper, B. (1978). Fundamental patterns of knowing in nursing. *Advances in Nursing Science, 1*(1), 13–23.

Carper, B. (1979). The ethics of caring. *Advances in Nursing Science, 1*(2), 11–19.

Chinn, P., & Jacobs, M. (1991). *Theory and nursing—A systematic approach.* St. Louis: C. V. Mosby.

Cronin, S. N., & Harrison, B. (1988). Importance of nurse caring behaviors as perceived by patients after myocardial infarction. *Heart and Lung, 17*(4), 374–380.

Daly, M. (1984). *Pure lust.* Boston: Beacon Press.

Diers, D. (1990). The art and craft of nursing. *American Journal of Nursing, 90*(1), 64–66.

Dunlap, M. (1986). Is a science of caring possible? *Journal of Advanced Nursing, 11*, 661–670.

Fawcett, J. (1984). The metaparadigm of nursing: Present status and future refinements. *Image: The Journal of Nursing Scholarship, 16*(3), 84–87.

Forest, D. (1989). The "experience" of caring. *Journal of Advanced Nursing, 14*, 815–823.

Gadow, S. (1979). Advocacy nursing and new meanings of aging. *Nursing Clinics of North America, 14*(1), 81–91.

Gadow, S. (1980). A model for ethical decision making. *Oncology Nursing Forum, 7*(4), 44–47.

Gadow, S. (1981). Truth: treatment of choice, scarce resource or patient's right? *The Journal of Family Practice, 13*(6), 857–860.

Gardner, D. (1985). Presence. In G. Bulechek, J. McCloskey, & M. Aydelotte (Eds.), *Nursing interventions—Treatment for nursing diagnoses.* Philadelphia: W. B. Saunders, 316–324.

Grove, P. B. (Ed.) (1963). *Webster's third new international dictionary.* Springfield, MA: G&C Merriam Co.

Heidegger, M. (1987). *An introduction to metaphysics.* New Haven: Yale University Press.

Hinds, P. S., Martin, J., & Vogel, R. J. (1987). Nursing strategies to influence adolescent hopefulness during oncologic illness. *Journal of Associated Pediatric Nurses, 4*(2), 14–22.

Hudson, R. (1988, September–November). Whole or parts—A theological perspective on "person." *The Australian Journal of Advanced Nursing, 6*(1), 20.

Johnson, M. (1980, January 7). Self disclosure: A variable in the nurse-client relationship. *Journal of Psychiatric Nursing and Mental Health Services.*

Larson, P. (1987). Comparisons of cancer patients' and professional nurses' perceptions of important nurse caring behaviors. *Heart and Lung,* 16(2), 187–192.

Leininger, M. M. (1986, July). Care facilitation and resistance factors in the culture of nursing. *Topics in Clinical Nursing,* 1–10.

Leonard, V. (1989). A Heideggerian phenomenologic perspective on the concept of person. *Advances in Nursing Science, 11*(4), 40–50.

Liehr, P. (1989). The core of true presence: A loving center. *Nursing Science Quarterly, 2,* 7–8.

Mayer, D. K. (1986). Cancer patients and families' perceptions of nurse caring behaviors. *Topics in Clinical Nursing,* 8(2), 63–69.

Merriam-Webster, A. (1988). *Webster's collegiate thesaurus.* Springfield, MA: Merriam-Webster, Inc.

Munhall, P., & Oiler, C. (1987). Language and nursing research. In P. Munhall, & C. Oiler, *Nursing research—A qualitative perspective.* Norwalk, CT: Appleton-Century-Croft, 3–25.

Newman, M. (1986). *Health as expanding consciousness.* St. Louis: C. V. Mosby.

Norris, C. (1984). *Concept clarification in nursing.* Rockville, MO: Aspen.

Parse, R. R. (1981). *Man-living-health: A theory of nursing.* New York: John Wiley & Sons.

Patterson, J., & Zderad, L. (1988). *Humanistic nursing.* New York: National League for Nursing.

Prager, E. (1989). A visit from the footbinder. In C. Park & C. Heaton (Ed.) *Close company: Stories of mothers and daughters.* New York: Ticknon & Fields, 48–76.

Quinn, J. F. (1984). The healing arts in modern health care. *The American Theosophist, 72*(5), 198–208.

Quinn, J. F. (1988). Building a body of knowledge: Research on therapeutic touch. *Journal of Holistic Nursing, 6*(1), 37–45.

Riemen, D. (1986). Noncaring and caring in the clinical setting: Patients' perceptions. *Topics in Clinical Nursing,* 8(2), 30–36.

Roach, Sr. M. S. (1987). *The human art of caring.* Ottawa: Canadian Hospital Association.

Rogers, M. (1981). Science of unitary man. In G. Lasker (Ed.), *A paradigm for nursing.* New York: Pergamon Press, 1719–1722.

Scarry, E. (1985). *The body in pain. The making and unmaking of the world.* New York: Oxford University Press.

Swanson-Kauffman, K. (1986). Caring in the instance of unexpected early pregnancy loss. *Topics in Clinical Nursing,* 8(2), 37–46.

The Oxford unabridged dictionary (1961). Oxford: The Clarendon Press.

Travelbee, J. (1971). *Interpersonal aspects of nursing.* Philadelphia: F. A. Davis Co.

Walker, L., & Avant, K. (1983). *Strategies for theory construction in nursing.* Norwalk, CT: Appleton & Lange, 35–49.

Watson, J. (1985). *Nursing: Human science and human care.* New York: National League for Nursing.

Watson (1989). Watson's Philosophy and Theory of Human Caring in Nursing. In R. Sisca (Ed.), *Conceptual models for nursing practice.* Appleton & Lange, 219–244.

Wheeler, C., & Chinn, P. (1989). *Peace and power.* New York: National League for Nursing.

Wilson, H. (1986). Presencing—Social control of schizophrenics in an antipsychiatric community: Doing grounded theory. In P. Munhall, & C. Oiler. *Nursing research—A qualitative perspective.* Norwalk, CT: Appleton-Century-Croft, 131–144.

Wilson, H. S. (1982). *Deinstitutionalized residential care for the mentally disordered—The Soteria house approach.* New York: Greene & Stratton.

Wilson, J. (1969). *Thinking with concepts.* London: Cambridge University Press.

5

The Caring Nursing Environment

Linda Dietrich

Recently literature on the nature and concept of caring has been proliferating. It is clear that caring is becoming viewed as a core component of the practice of nursing (Leininger, 1984; Watson, 1979). Caring can be viewed as an affect, a human trait, moral imperative, interpersonal interaction, or a therapeutic intervention (Morse et al., 1990). Benner & Wrubel (1989) discuss, "If nurses are to liberate caring practices, organizations will have to be redesigned to facilitate and sponsor caring practices" (p. 399). Many studies have described the caring relationship between nurses and patients (Brown, 1986; Weiss, 1988; Wolf, 1986; Benner, 1984; Benner & Wrubel, 1989). Unfortunately little attention has been placed on understanding the concept of caring in nurse-nurse interactions in the work environment, the settings where the art of nursing is practiced. If the same emphasis was applied to nursing interactions in the work setting, perhaps greater individual and professional satisfaction would result in the practice environment.

To facilitate and sponsor caring practices within the acute care nursing work environment, it is important to uncover and describe what these caring practices are. This study describes the caring practices, experiences, and meanings of nurse-nurse caring, non-caring, and arrangements and structures in the environment that promote or inhibit caring within the context of a 33-bed neurovascular acute care nursing unit.

LITERATURE REVIEW

Provision of caring in the nursing environment is considered facilitative of quality caring practices. Shiber & Larson (1991) express that caregivers cannot impart caring unless they are cared for themselves or are part of a caring environment. The environment with which the care provider interacts during the process of giving care is connected with care recipients' health outcomes. Kayser-Jones (1991) has linked physical, psychosocial, and organizational features of the environment to quality of care for the elderly. Valentine (1989) structurally conceptualized the process of caring between nurses and patients in an acute care nursing context, utilizing nurses, clients, and nurse theorist/researchers. Using a naturalistically based mixed-method approach, Valentine (1991) identified relationships between the context and process of caring and selected health outcomes of clients.

Caring cannot be viewed apart from the environment in which it occurs. Ray (1989) addressed the meaning of caring in the hospital culture and identified that how caring was defined and practiced within nursing units was determined by the unit context. The majority of American nurses continue to practice within the context of the acute care nursing environment or hospital setting (Moses, 1990). In the hospital setting, the nurse is in constant interaction with patients and colleagues. Shiber & Larson (1991) have described the availability of a nurse colleague reference group that supports a caring environment which serves as a structure in the organization that supports caring.

DESIGN

In the present study, I used a naturalistic approach. According to Patton (1987), the naturalistic approach assumes phenomena are contextual, emerging, and unique and offers an interpretation of phenomena through the meaning it has to others. I chose a naturalistic approach because of the contextual nature of caring and the importance of delineating descriptions of caring based upon interpretations and meanings from staff nurses.

SAMPLE AND METHOD

In-depth tape recorded open-ended interviews on a purposive sample of five registered nurses were done over a two-week period of time. Three shifts were represented. The age range of the study participants was 29 to 54 years. All five were female. Experience as a registered nurse ranged from 6 to 33 years and length of time on the neurovascular unit was 5 to 16 years. To enhance building trust and learning the culture, meetings with the staff on two different occasions to explain the study and how the results would be used were conducted. Participation in the study was voluntary, informed consent was obtained prior to interviews, and anonymity and confidentiality were guaranteed by the researcher. An interview guide constructed to elicit meanings of nurse-nurse caring and non-caring and structures and arrangements in the environment that supported or inhibited caring, was used to facilitate the interview. An open-ended format and intent toward abeyance of values and interpretations on the part of the interviewer during sessions enhanced the probability of credible findings.

ANALYSIS

The interview data were coded using the phenomenologic method. Through a process of structured reflection on the nurses' expressions of their caring experiences descriptive themes were discovered. To assure internal consistency and mutual exclusivity of each theme, coding and content analysis was done on five separate occasions. Central themes and dimensions of experiences which evolved from the data analysis are described below. Texts in quotations are derived directly from interview data. The expressions of the nurses' caring experiences are arranged under four perspectives: Nurse-Nurse Caring, Nurse-Nurse Non-Caring, Arrangements or Structures in the Environment that Promote Caring, and Arrangements or Structures in the Environment that Inhibit Caring.

FINDINGS

Nurse-Nurse Caring

Table 1 describes the meanings of nurse-nurse caring expressed by the respondents. Meanings were clustered into seven themes.

Theme 1: Being Sensitive. Awareness of what other nurses are going through who are involved in similar work develops through personal life experience. Such awareness may express itself as sensitivity to coworkers' responses and management of their workloads. Expressing concern about a coworker's workload is perceived as caring.

> *You're aware of what the other nurses are going through. All I have to do is look at a face to be able to tell if they're harassed or worried about something. You can be sensitive enough to know what's happening.*

> *I think most nurses are sensitive to someone rushing about, or getting a lot of calls. I think everybody is aware of what kind of day it is that one another is having.*

> *They just need to say: "How are you doing with your load? Do you feel you can care for another patient right now?"*

> *If they are giving me another patient, they might ask: "How is your workload? How are you doing with the workload that you have?"*

> *I'm not sure they (nurses) may not start with it. It may be something that they have to learn as they get on because once you are into it and you are aware of what you're going through, then you are sensitive to what other people are going through also.*

Table 1
Nurse-Nurse Caring

Theme 1: Being Sensitive
Being sensitive is being aware of others around you, how things are affecting them and what kind of a work day they are having.
Sensitivity develops through knowledge of other nurses' experience.
Knowledge is acquired through personal first-hand experience.

Theme 2: Offering Help
Offering help is being available to offer assistance to other nurses with patient care and is limited by the realities of the practice setting such as time and workloads.

Theme 3: Being Open
Being open is taking things with an open mind.
Being open-minded means listening to another.

Theme 4: Being Understanding
Being understanding is responding in a sympathetic and tolerant manner.

Theme 5: Acknowledgement
Acknowledgement of a coworker's knowledge and skill and making them feel that "they made a difference."
Acknowledging a coworker's presence, and recognizing them as a whole person.

Theme 6: Being Supportive
Being supportive is carrying the load for another nurse.
Being supportive is comforting.
Being supportive is not causing someone to feel guilty for calling in ill.
Being supportive is responding in an honest and consistent manner and builds trust and a sense of team.

Theme 7: Camaraderie
Camaraderie is a sense of fellowship or "We are all in this together."

Theme 2: Offering Help. Showing concern for another nurse's workload by offering help is a luxury.

Many times I am aware that someone needs help but I don't have the luxury to offer assistance because I am in dire straits myself.

It is infrequent that I am caught up enough to actually seek people out and say: "Do you need some help, what can I do for you?"

Theme 3: Being Open. Being broad-minded enough to listen to a coworker's view and to convey to another coworker that you are listening is perceived as caring.

I think it's the worse thing one can do is to not listen to someone else's point of view, or opinion. If you don't agree with it, take it with an open mind.

The totally closed mind is wrong. It doesn't accomplish anything. It causes bad feelings and hurts relationships.

Just listen to me or let me feel like I am being listened to. If I have an explanation or a feeling. If they can just let me know they're listening to me.

To listen if there is a problem or have a question about something I have done. To be aware enough to listen for other peoples' problems.

Theme 4: Being Understanding.   Being sympathetic and patient in interactions with coworkers experiencing either personal or professional problems can be perceived as caring.

Sometimes you don't want to pry into their personal lives so you don't ask why they (nurse coworkers) are grumpy. You back away and help where you need to. I suppose a way of sharing or caring is to let them not share.

When mistakes are made with patient care don't immediately say, "You messed up, I'm going to report you because you messed up!"

Theme 5: Acknowledgement.   Appreciating a coworker for his or her knowledge and skills and valuing him or her as a whole person shows caring.

If someone has handled a situation well or stood their ground while having difficulty with a doctor, tell them that they did a good job, or you did very well, or try to pat them on the back or some kind of contact.

Just telling each other, "You did a good job. You taught me something."

Letting you feel that you made a difference.

We need to keep in touch with each other throughout the workday on a regular basis. We have to talk about personal things in nursing. Otherwise it gets to be like you just come in and do your time.

Be concerned for coworkers other than just in the work environment. Take an interest in their life outside. Try to get to know them as complete persons instead of nurses you work with.

Theme 6: Being Supportive. Showing concern for another nurse when he or she is unable to carry workload due to illness or personal reasons is a way of showing caring and creates a supportive atmosphere and enhances trust. Likewise, when honest, consistent information regarding patient care is given from peers, the environment is perceived as supportive, building trust and a sense of team.

Everybody flocked around and tried to be supportive of me and tried to give me a break to gather myself together. They were just there for me and covered for me as I tried to pull my life back together for 30 or 40 minutes.

If someone is stressed out and has been taking care of a particularly difficult patient for several days, just having someone take over that patient.

If I ask someone about a medication or physiology or something significant about a patient, I know they won't lead me astray. If they don't know, they will tell me they don't know. If I need help with something, I know they will help me.

Theme 7: Camaraderie. *Esprit de corps* develops as a nurse becomes part of a unique nursing community. Respecting this sense of community esprit de corps is a way of showing caring.

It's a kind of camaraderie. It's not really a specific action, but I know enough about where I work that how we show we care for each other is just a feeling of needing.

Trying to make them understand that something that happened to them has happened to other nurses.

Being able to make light of a particularly busy or difficult day.

Nurse-Nurse Non-Caring

Table 2 describes the meanings of nurse-nurse non-caring expressed by respondents. Meanings were clustered into three themes discussed below.

Theme 1: Lack of Respect. Inconsiderate confrontation (or lack of a confrontation) regarding patient care issues is perceived as non-caring. In the same sense, lack of deference for another's knowledge and skills is perceived as non-caring. A nurse can feel a lack of respect and non-caring when thoughtfulness and tact are lacking during confrontations regarding mistakes made with patient care.

> *If I tried to say I'm sorry this mistake was made, I was told it shouldn't have been made. I tried to explain I would be more careful the next time. The response I got was this: "The mistake shouldn't have been made in the first place."*

> *There are times when I make mistakes. I am human, and just because I am a nurse doesn't mean I am not allowed to make mistakes.*

> *There is no more discussion than you made a mistake, you messed up, and that is the big thing. It makes me feel they aren't*

Table 2
Nurse–Nurse Non-Caring

Theme 1: Lack of Respect
    Lack of respect occurs when another nurse is denied the right to be human and make mistakes.
    Lack of respect occurs when a nurse is not confronted about mistakes in a sensitive and open manner.
    Lack of respect for another's knowledge and skills.

Theme 2: Lack of Acknowledgement
    Not being acknowledged is floating to another unit and no one tells you that they're glad you're there.
    One can have a sense of lack of acknowledgement by administration.
    Lack of acknowledgement is when you perceive you are being ignored by your peers or administration in relation to plans or standards of patient care.

Theme 3: Lack of Camaraderie
    Lack of camaraderie is purposely setting a negative tone for the day.
    Lack of camaraderie is not cooperating with coworkers.

trusting me any more. I don't want to come to work. I don't feel I'm being trusted by them. I feel hurt and insulted, like my intelligence was insulted, my competency insulted, like I had the inability to make a judgment.

I think being up front with someone and sharing with them that there is a problem with patient care is better than talking about that person's behavior. Caring can be sharing with someone why you are upset, and what you would like them to do to improve.

Many times it is in the tone with which things are said, such as in a harsh or critical manner. If someone could just say, look, here is a better way I learned . . .

People can talk to each other on the same level or a person can talk to another person in a downward manner. A downward manner conveys the perception: I know what I'm doing, but you don't so let me tell you how to do it. People don't like to work on a unit that conveys a critical attitude.

Theme 2: Lack of Acknowledgement. When a nurse's contribution is not acknowledged or valued by others or when plans regarding patient care are ignored by peers it can be perceived as non-caring.

It is more of a general sense from the CEO on down that administration is a step removed from the experience of dealing with the patient. Yet how the patient perceives his or her stay is related to how well I am able to manage my workload and how well I am able to get care to this or that person. Sometimes you don't know if they really understand what you are doing.

When people from administration come around and ask you how things are going and you tell them it's really terrible, they really don't care so why did they ask.

My perception may be ignored by the previous nurses. That in a sense makes me feel not cared for. If I don't do it, no one else is going to do it. I better do everything while I am here because I don't know if the next person is going to do it.

I feel I am not cared for when I feel there were things I left undone, or not properly done or just not up to snuff.

I feel that I have very high standards and I do my best to meet all my patients' needs. I believe that nurses should come to work on time, do their work, and get out on time. While they are at work they need to concentrate on getting their work done, on not fooling around, on not being inappropriate with family and things like that. So I guess that when people are not doing what they are supposed to, I see it as not being caring.

Theme 3: Lack of Camaraderie. When the *esprit de corps* of the group is not respected, it is perceived as non-caring.

When somebody says to you it's going to be a terrible day, that sets the tone for the day. It adds stress to walk on the unit. You hear it when they call for nine staff and there are only seven on duty.

The thing that I hate is when you come on shift and they say, "If you knew what was good for you, you'd go back home."

It is part of your job to have good interactions with coworkers. If you aren't caring and can't cooperate or work with other people, then you can't do a good job and care for your patients because it carries through to everything you do.

Arrangements or Structures in the Environment That Promote Caring

Table 3 describes the environmental factors perceived as promoting caring as expressed by the respondents. Meanings were clustered into one theme.

Support of Nursing Management. Nurses perceived the following arrangements and structures as promoting caring in their environment.

Table 3
Arrangements or Structures in the
Environment That Promote Caring

Theme: Support of Nursing Management

Nursing management that promotes communication is perceived as being supportive and by being available and visible, on a daily and consistent basis and being easy to talk to.

Nursing management that allows time to ask questions and vent concerns.

Hospital offerings such as conferences and Nurses Day make you feel that they are at least feeling about you.

A clear organizational mission integrated to the unit level.

I like having administrative people just show up on the unit unannounced and walk around. Being able to access a person one to one is important.

Being able to see nursing administration in an informal setting is important, not having to ask a question in front of 50 people.

Nursing management should allow time to ask questions and vent concerns.

Hospital offerings such as conferences and Nurses Day make you feel that they are at least feeling about you.

I think there is more caring now because everyone receives the information about the hospital mission in orientation and every year the statement is reviewed by the staff.

Arrangements or Structures in the Environment That Inhibit Caring

Table 4 describes the environmental factors in the environment perceived as inhibiting caring as expressed by the respondents. Meanings were clustered into two themes.

Theme 1: Interactions. Opportunities to interact apart from direct patient care and develop caring relationships is limited.

Table 4
Arrangements or Structures in the
Environment That Inhibit Caring

Theme 1: Interactions
  The lack of interaction between nurses on different shifts.
  Lack of time and space to interact away from direct patient care.

Theme 2: Perception of the Workload
  When workloads are perceived as being overwhelming, nurses feel like they
  can't do their job because there simply isn't enough time or help. It is emotionally and physically draining and can result in a sense of hopelessness or
  system overload from the overall scheme of things.
  The availability of help in a timely manner makes the workload easier to deal
  with.

Sometimes unit parties end up being shift parties. It would be nice to do things as a group instead of being intershifted.

There is no place to congregate with any kind of privacy and pull back for a few minutes and sink into a chair. There is very little time. You need time to be with your peers and be able to talk, be away from the patients and their families and talk about your patients if you need to and relax for a little while, and you can't always do that in the cafeteria.

We communicate with each other when we turn patients, get them in and out of bed, or up to the commode. Usually, we each have a patient that we require help from another nurse to give care to.

You need a place to rest from all the work, physical activity, and mental activity that is involved with nursing care.

Theme 2: Perception of the Workload. The way a nurse perceives his or her workload influences the experience of the environment as caring or non-caring.

Just being overworked to the point where you feel like you can't do your job as safely as it should be done, and then I feel more not cared for by the hospital. How can you do this to me, put me in this position where I can't give them the kind of care I want to. Just feeling frustrated . . .

Table 5
Caring Concepts and Supportive Strategies

Categorical Data	To Increase Caring in the Work Environment
Being sensitive	Increase awareness of others.
Offering help	Clarify workload issues.
Being open	Promote active listening.
Being understanding	Promote sympathy and tolerance.
Acknowledgement	Peer and administrative recognition.
Being supportive	Promote consistent, honest communication.
Camaraderie	Articulate a sense of fellowship.
Respecting others	Encourage an atmosphere of risk taking and considerate confrontation.
Interactions	Promote interactions between shifts.
	Create time and spaces for nurses to interact apart from direct client care.
Support of nursing management	Clear, consensual standards of care integrated at the bedside level.
	Nursing management available, visible, and easy to talk to.
	Formal and informal recognition of nurses.
Workloads	Clarify work to be done; expectations; standards of care to be met based on resources.
	Provide help in a timely manner if possible.

Coming in and having the patient tell you that such and such didn't happen since yesterday and maybe I'd made a point of saying to my peers you need to do this for the patient. It goes back to everybody's amount of time. I trust them and their ability as workers. It comes back to a time factor, they just don't have enough time.

System overload: It's really not related to any particular person, but just the overall scheme of things. It makes you feel physically and emotionally pooped.

The availability of help in a timely manner makes the workload easier to deal with.

Table 5 presents a summary of the categorical data (column 1). Strategies to increase caring within the environment (column 2) are suggested based on study data and interpretations of the researcher. A discussion of the interpretations follows.

Discussion

Themes emerged that are consistent with other authors' descriptions of caring processes embodied within the relationship between nurse and client. Caring was identified as an interpersonal relationship, therapeutic intervention, affect, human trait, and moral imperative.

Caring as an Interpersonal Interaction or Therapeutic Intervention. The nurse-nurse caring and non-caring categories have elements relative to the work of those who view caring as an interpersonal relationship. The learned experience of nurses caring for other nurses through living within the same contextual reality is synonymous to Benner and Wrubel's (1989) descriptions of the connectedness of being in caring encounters. Weiss (1988) described verbal and non-verbal behaviors present in the ideal nurse-client caring situation such as addressing the patient with respect (verbal) and attending to the patient or making oneself available to the patient using active or attentive listening (non-verbal). Similarly, the nurses' descriptions of feeling "not cared for" when not being confronted about mistakes in a respectful manner (verbal) or the perception of caring as being listening with an open mind (non-verbal) are similar to those described by Weiss.

If, as described by Gaut (1986), caring is a mediated action, then the ability to interact would be a prerequisite for caring to occur. When there is lack of time and space to interact away from direct patient care and lack of interaction between shifts, this can inhibit caring in the nurse work-group environment. Specific actions such as openness, active listening, and attempting to know another nurse as a whole person, enable caring to occur in the nurse-nurse relationship. Valentine (1989) and Wolf (1986) also refer to openness and active or attentive listening as elements of caring interventions in the nurse-client relationship.

Affect. According to Bevis (1981), acting without instant recognition for acts is a component of caring. McFarlane (1976) discussed that elements of protection and oversight are embodied in caring. The images of caring as an affect are exemplified in the themes of nurse-nurse caring as being understanding and supportive.

Human Trait.   In another study, dominant descriptors of caring
on medical surgical units were associated with teamwork. According
to Ray (1989), activities involved in providing caring services to patients are affected by competition for scarce resources. Similarly, *context* significantly influenced how caring was defined and practiced in
the environment of the neurovascular unit. Offering help to coworkers with patient care, being supportive by carrying the load for
another nurse when necessary, and the aspect of camaraderie appeared as descriptors indicative of a sense of team as caring. Learn
caring is exemplified by one respondent who said, "We always have a
patient where we need another nurse's help to care for that patient."
This also supports the context-dependent nature of caring. The
salient meaning of caring within the bureaucratic habitat of an acute
care hospital nursing unit may be a crucial indicator for nursing administrators interested in assessing environmental needs and culture.

Moral Imperative.   Cognitive dissonance occurs when a nurse
attempts to be caring in an incongruent environment. Some nurses
discussed the acceptability of mistakes in regard to patient care.
Others reflected upon concerns regarding time and resource limitations and what realistically can be done for clients in an acute care
setting. Morals indicate what we value. Perhaps manifestations of
"system overload" and responses of being physically and emotionally
exhausted in relation to the overall scheme of things is connected to
such cognitive dissonance.

Since one nurse may value caring aspects of practice more than
another, this may cause conflicting values over clinical decisions
regarding care delivery. Such conflict is exemplified by the nurse
who stated, "I guess that when people are not doing what they are
supposed to I see as not being caring."

Implications to Practice

The workload of patient care as an arrangement or structure in
the environment that influences caring permeates the descriptions
given by nurses. The perception of patient care workload intensity is
a common thread that pervaded all categories. Within the themes of

nurse-nurse caring, being sensitive and aware of a coworker's response to their workload, the luxury of being able to offer help with patient care, being understanding when mistakes are made in regard to patient care, supporting a peer by helping with their workload, and camaraderie unfolded as a shared feeling of needing each other in order to effectively manage the workload.

Similarly, within the nurse-nurse non-caring category, lack of respect occurs when nurses are denied the right to be human and make mistakes in providing patient care or when they are not confronted about those mistakes in a considerate and timely manner. In the same sense, lack of acknowledgement regarding standards of patient care by peers has direct implications to perception of the environment as caring or non-caring.

As long as the focus of nursing in the acute care environment continues to be on the medically delegated dependent aspects of practice, the perception of workload will be driven by this perspective. However, a key to transforming this perspective and managing the issue of workload intensity perception may be in delineating what the work is that needs to be done in caring for patients. Developing clear consensual standards of care that focus on the independent caring aspects of nursing care integrated into the realities of daily practice is one strategy for delineating and clarifying care expectations in the work setting. The Clinical Practice Model developed by Wesorick (1991) uses such a strategy. This model may decrease the cognitive dissonance of nurses who want to practice the art of caring in a bureaucratic environment.

If practice standards are unclear and nonconsensual, nurses may create unrealistic expectations or assumptions about what should or can be accomplished in the course of a workday. Consequently, a sense of feeling overloaded or overworked, or that a nurse must get everything done in eight hours, can occur since nurses commonly perceive they cannot trust the next nurse to do it. Because personal standards may be used to judge the acceptability of mistakes regarding patient care, an atmosphere can occur in which nurses perceive a lack of understanding, openness, and trust from their peers.

Many nursing organizations in the acute care hospital environment have written standards of care in place. However, simply having written standards may not be sufficient. The process of creating explicit, consensual, realistic practice standards based on organizational resources available to deliver the standards may need to be considered. Additionally, integrating nursing care standards into each component of daily practice by providing resources and tools for the bedside practitioner facilitates accountable caring practice. Decisions and conflicts regarding workload issues based on explicit standards versus implicit standards provide a structure for basic practice accountability. When expectations regarding the work of caring for patients are clarified and agreed upon by the work group, then it becomes clear what each practitioner is accountable for and what he or she holds peers accountable for.

The way nurses are able to interact within the practice setting also was identified as a factor that inhibited caring in the environment. Nursing administrators might consider promoting interactions between nurses as a unit instead of nurses within shifts and providing time and space for interactions between nurses apart from direct patient care. Nursing management being visible, available, and approachable on a consistent daily basis was identified as an arrangement or structure in the environment that promoted caring. Hospital offerings such as Nurses Day, conferences, and the director of nursing's monthly meetings with employees also were mentioned by participants as being supportive.

CONCLUSION

Nursing administrators, researchers, and practitioners have an important role in supporting the development and implementation of caring practice models for professionals who practice the art of caring in institutional settings. Further studies that describe the concept of caring in the nurse's work setting can assist in the development of strategies to support caring processes in the nursing work environment. This knowledge is needed by nurse administrators and practitioners if organizations are to be redesigned to sponsor and promote caring. Perhaps by increasing the congruency between the nurse and her environment, greater individual and professional realization of caring in the practice setting of the acute care hospital can be realized.

REFERENCES

Benner, P. (1984). *From novice to expert excellence and power in clinical nursing practice.* Menlo Park, CA: Addison-Wesley.

Benner, P., & Wrubel, J. (1989). *The primacy of caring stress and coping in health and illness.* Menlo Park, CA: Addison-Wesley.

Bevis, E. O. (1981). Caring: A life force. In M. M. Leininger (Ed.), *Caring: An essential human need. Proceedings of the three national caring conferences.* Thorofare, NJ: Slack, 49–59.

Brown, L. (1986). The experience of care: Patient perspectives. *Topics in Clinical Nursing, 8*(2), 56–62.

Gaut, D. (1986). Evaluating caring competencies in nursing. *Topics in Clinical Nursing, 8,* 77–83.

Kayser-Jones, J. S. (1991). The impact of the environment on the quality of care in nursing homes: A social psychological perspective. *Holistic Nursing Practice, 5*(3), 29–38.

Leininger, M. M. (Ed.) (1984). *Care: The essence of nursing and health.* Thorofare, NJ: Slack.

McFarlane, J. (1976). A charter for caring. *Journal of Advanced Nursing, 1,* 187–196.

Morse, J. M., Solberg, S. M., Neander, W. L., Botoroff, J. L., & Johnston, J. L. (1990). Concepts of caring and caring as concept. *Advances in Nursing Science, 13*(1), 1–14.

Moses, E. B. (1990). Profile of the contemporary nursing population: Findings from the 1988 sample survey of registered nurses data sources. In *Perspectives in nursing—1989–1991.* New York. National League for Nursing, 33–44.

Patton, M. (1987). *How to use qualitative methods in evaluation.* Newbury Park, CA: Sage.

Ray, M. (1989). The theory of bureaucratic caring for nursing practice in the organizational culture. *Nursing Administration Quarterly, 13*(2), 31–42.

Shiber, S., & Larson, E. (1991). Evaluating the quality of caring: Structure, process, and outcome. *Holistic Nursing Practice, 5*(3), 57–66.

Valentine, K. (1989). Contributions to the theory of care. *Evaluation and Program Planning, 12*(1), 17–23.

Valentine, K. (1991). Comprehensive assessment of caring and its relationship to outcome measures. *Journal of Nursing Quality Assurance, 5*(2), 59–68.

Watson, J. (1979). *Nursing: The philosophy and science of caring.* Boston: Little, Brown.

Weiss, C. J. (1988). Model to discover validate and use care in nursing. In M. M. Leininger (Ed.), *Care: Discovery and uses in clinical and community nursing*. Detroit: Wayne State University Press, 139–149.

Wesorick, B. (1991). Creating an environment in the hospital setting that supports caring via a clinical practice model (CPM). In D. Gaut & M. M. Leininger (Ed.), *Caring the compassionate healer*. New York. National League for Nursing, 135–160.

Wolf, Z. R. (1986). The caring concept and nurse identified caring behaviors. *Topics in Clinical Nursing, 8*(2), 84–93.

6

Reflections on the Promotion of Caring with Head Nurses

Suzanne Kerouac
Lesley Rouillier

In this article, we describe the process and findings of a participative research study designed to enable a group of head nurses to promote caring in their practice. Through eight group sessions with one author acting as a facilitator, the group discussed and explored the caring components of clinical and administrative nursing. A theoretical statement emerges from this experience.

INTRODUCTION

In Canada, as in the United States, the bureaucratic and technological environment of today's health care institutions has relegated the human character of care and caring to the background. For those who seek to promote professional caring, this situation causes considerable concern. The constant undermining and undervaluing of the very *raison d'être* of the nursing profession have negative effects on both nurses and nursing practice. Low recruitment, high turnover, burnout, and lack of competent nursing care are indications of those effects (Baumgart & Larsen, 1988; Benner & Wrubel, 1989; Harris, 1989; Leininger, 1988a,b; Order of Nurses of Québec, 1989; Québec Hospital Association, 1988; Ray, 1988b; Roach, 1984, 1987; Watson, 1988).

Under present conditions, support from both colleagues and superiors is required if the clinical staff's caring endeavours are to be sustained. Studies by Harris (1984), Hillestad (1984), and Scalzi (1988) show that practicing nurse administrators feel unsupported and lonely and that they experience role stress. Furthermore, they often are perceived as being different from their clinical colleagues. Many clinicians are of the opinion that once a nurse assumes an administrative role, the dynamic aspects of his or her nursing knowledge and practice are automatically neutralized.

The perceived separation of nurse administrators from nurse clinicians could be reduced by uniting the two around such common concepts as person, health, environment, and nursing (Jennings & Meleis, 1988). Another uniting force is found in Leininger's (1988c) statement that "caring is the unique, unifying, and dominant focus of nursing" (p. 83). The singular role of first-line nurse administrators (head nurses) includes such responsibilities as the practice of clinical nursing, the promotion of caring, and the creation of a conducive, healthy work environment (Christenson, 1988; Jennings & Meleis, 1988; Rowland & Rowland, 1985; Stevens, 1985). Although to become a caring person requires being treated in a caring way, this can be nurtured or inhibited by the environment (Gaylin, 1976; Marz, 1986; Mayeroff, 1971; Roach, 1984, 1987).

Based on the above considerations, the authors undertook a participative research project to enable a group of head nurses to promote caring in their practice. As defined, initial study assumptions included: (1) every person has the potential for growth; (2) growth is facilitated by caring behaviors; (3) among these caring behaviors, sharing, discussing, and learning are nurtured within a group; (4) group experiences are beneficial to head nurses; and (5) discussions on caring are both a learning and a supportive experience for head nurses.

REFERENCE FRAMEWORK

Among the various theories about caring, of significance for this study were Watson (1985a,b), Leininger (1980, 1988a,b,d), Roach (1984, 1987), Gaut (1983, 1986, 1988), and Ray (1987, 1988a,b, 1989).

While Watson's (1985a,b) theory of human science and human care focuses on the dynamic reciprocal transpersonal relationship between the client and the nurse, Leininger (1980, 1988a,b,c) emphasizes the influence of culture on these two actors in her theory of transcultural care and caring (Leininger, 1980, 1988a,b,c). Roach (1984, 1987), in describing five attributes of caring, underlines the importance of the experience of being cared for if one is to acquire the ability to care. Gaut's (1983, 1986, 1988) action description of caring—setting a goal, choosing a tactic, and implementing the tactic based on need and desired positive change—shows how these reciprocal actions are influenced by the context in which they are performed. Ray's (1987, 1988a,b, 1989) research in a hospital context shows that this organizational culture often affects caring negatively. She calls for the integration of a theory of caring into the clinical and administrative components of practice as a means of moulding the organizational cultural context into one of caring enhancement.

In the same vein, other experts in nursing agree that adherence to pure managerial theory is not well suited to the administration of nursing. These experts propose generating a theory for nursing administration focused on a synthesis of shared managerial and nursing concepts. Here, concerns for nursing personnel, promotion of nursing values, and the creation of a favorable climate for nursing practice are the foundations of the development of a nursing administration theory (Benner & Wrubel, 1989; Blair, 1989; Chaska, 1983; Christenson, 1988; Dunham, 1989; Jennings, 1987; Jennings & Meleis, 1988; Miller, 1987; Nyberg, 1989; Stevens, 1983).

Some believe that caring is a unifying link between administrative and clinical nursing practice. They propose that nurse managers—directors of nursing, head nurses, as well as those at other administrative levels—exemplify caring by the consistent development of caring behaviors within their administrative activities

(Benner & Wrubel, 1989; Dunham, 1989; Jennings, 1987; and Nyberg, 1989).

As suggested, individual learning and behavioral change can be provided within a group experience (Barrett-Lennard, 1975; Claus & Bailey, 1977; Culbert, 1975; Hogue, Levesque, & Morin, 1988; Lakin & Costanzo, 1975; Lieberman, Yalom, & Miles, 1973; Rogers, 1970; Schutz, 1966; Yalom, 1985). The fostering of interpersonal communications and participation establishes the support necessary for efficient task accomplishment and the attainment of organizational or social goals, thus promoting organizational health.

Interactions within a group and, consequently, group outcomes, can be positively influenced by facilitative leadership (Lieberman, Yalom, & Miles, 1973; Rogers, 1970). A facilitator trusts the group to develop at its own rhythm and according to its own potential, allows the group to develop its own direction, and permits the expression of the whole person, whether oneself or the other, in both cognitive and affect modes.

PROJECT DESIGN

In the present project, the head nurses and I, the facilitator, worked together to establish the focus, guidelines, process, and outcomes of the experience within a nursing administration focus. Guiding the evolution of the project (Gaut, 1983, 1988) were guidelines of a caring action, such as setting a goal, choosing a tactic and implementing it according to the need and the desire for change. I met with the director of nursing and the head nurses from a surgical nursing division to inform them of the project and to request their consent. Willingness to participate was the criterion for inclusion in the group. Five head nurses, all women, were invited and agreed to participate. Because I was "a stranger" to these women, to use Leininger's (1985) expression, I met privately with each head nurse several times to get acquainted, I also spent several hours as a participant observer becoming familiar with the nursing units and the hospital milieu.

PROJECT EVOLUTION

The project evolved through eight two-hour group encounters held from March to June 1990. Initially, in response to my question, "Tell me in your own words what caring means to you," several views emerged: "Caring is subjectivity, putting yourself in the other's position. It is subtleties, nonverbal, and verbal meanings: depends upon the patient's perceptions. It takes time and energy. It's liking what you're doing, it's more than just tasks, it's openness to others, offering help, addressing fears. It's related to the needs of the bedside nurse, her needs to be cared for."

These views enabled a preliminary exploration of the previously identified philosophies, premises, and definitions; all strong influences on the participants' work as caregivers throughout project evolution. We were reminded of the depth and the richness of the caring paradigm and, from daily critical events, received the impetus to include those values in our discussions. We became aware that the components of caring are a common ground for bedside and head nurses who share the same concerns for patients' well being and for quality of care. The one who cares for others needs to be cared for herself or himself. The following from a head nurse participant especially illustrates this point:

A dying patient was suddenly transferred to our unit this morning. As I entered his room, I saw the nurse desperately trying to initiate urgent nursing procedures while an angry family member, the patient's son, was yelling at her. The nurse, a mild-mannered girl, looked frustrated and answered him curtly. I remembered our group discussions about the expression of feelings and, turning to the son, I said softly: You seem very angry! He calmed down right away, acknowledging that it was exactly how he felt. I then said, "What is happening?" He told me his story. Afterwards, the nurse came to me and asked, "How did you manage that? Thank you!" I explained to her what I had done and why. I had been worried that she would feel that I was taking over. But she needed help; I could tell from the way she was acting. The family needed help

*too. By being a role model, I know that I was able to teach this
nurse without any loss of self-esteem on her part.*

By the fourth encounter, participant interactions involved sharing
of knowledge, self-expression, feedback, showing confidence in the
other, humor, and the resolution, by some, of a previous interpersonal conflict. These supporting behaviors continued outside of
group encounters as well.

Later on, we came to see how the roles of care giver and care
receiver evolve within a contractual relationship wherein there exists
a "fit": the care giver is able to identify and respond to the needs of
the care receiver, decoding his or her language and using his or her
strengths and abilities. The nurse is able to recognize differences
between personal values, perceptions, needs, and those of the oth-
er(s) involved. Working toward a common goal, using the strengths
and abilities of the care receiver, served to unite the two persons. The
relationship is energizing for the person who gives when that person
perceives recognition from the one who receives.

Our examination of cultural influences assisted in identifying
factors which promote or inhibit caring. We discussed how the
cultural patterns of the patient determine the caring processes as
well as why such processes must be identified, understood, and
considered by all involved. In addition, we saw that the nurse's
culture, including skills, gender, and personal obligations, influenced both practice and unit management. Relationships with
other health professionals also have an impact on caring abilities as
do institutional factors of organization, philosophies, use of technology, and change processes.

For these head nurses, therefore, integrating caring into nursing
practice meant getting to know the staff, appreciating their
strengths, and matching assignments accordingly. Other aspects
included sharing difficult situations, being a role model, and responding to the staff's needs expressed through staff behaviors.
Rewarding caring behaviors in a meaningful way also became an
important focus. Mixing the staff by affinities and skills dealt with
the importance of group work on the unit as did implementing
clear and realistic organizational changes according to the staff's

real needs. Participants' understanding of individual roles and responsibilities involved relationships with patients, health professionals, and the institution.

In my later encounters with project participants, which became more intense, they expressed immediate and positive feelings of trust, respect, confidence, and affection toward each other, and some negative feelings of sorrow, frustration, and anger associated with their administrative roles. Spontaneous, direct, personal feedback involving receptivity, reciprocity, and empathy was manifest. In this regard, the participants were able to identify and discuss their own needs of support from their nursing leaders.

As researcher, my caring actions towards the participants throughout project evolution included praise, acceptance, genuineness, sensitivity, concern, warmth, confidence, respect, and support. I exhibited praise and acceptance by validating their beliefs in their professional and administrative roles by sharing my own perceptions and experiences and comparing all these with pertinent literature. This also involved giving positive feedback, and showing my appreciation of their difficult situations. Genuineness encompassed honest open expression.

I expressed sensitivity to the focus at hand, an increased awareness, by increased observational and analytic abilities and by supportive verbal and nonverbal behaviors. I showed concern and warmth by taking care that all members were included in the discussions. I demonstrated confidence in and respect of participants by allowing them as a group and as individuals to develop their own rhythm, potential, and self-sufficiency as well as by my discretion and my willingness to accept confrontations as they arose. Other behaviors involved active listening, reformulating, asking open and contrasting questions, and doing content and process analysis. Also included were accepting the expressions of feelings, and relating these and other behaviors to the relevant caring literature.

Later, while reviewing and validating the content of the encounters, the head nurses related their real life experiences to the theories, commenting: "I see we didn't invent anything"; "I hadn't realized that all that was caring"; "Why don't they teach us this in school?"

FINDINGS

Outcomes of this experience were measured by the criterion of the welfare of the person for whom the action was carried out (Gaut, 1983, 1988). Numerous participants' views expressed immediate positive outcomes. Goal attainment also served as a second criterion to evaluate the success of the strategy; it was estimated by the degree to which the group discussions related to the reference framework.

During the project, the head nurse participants expressed their views of the experience.

> *I have restructured my thinking about nursing administration. It's team building, cohesion, taking into consideration the people within. It's being realistic in your expectations, and helping people to grow. We can contribute to the whole system by our actions.*
>
> *I got support from my peers, learned to accept support from my staff, I don't feel so lonely. We think a lot about caring and share it with the staff. I think about how to really support my staff, I ask them what their needs are. When we show an interest in what they do, the nurses feel valued that we care. The staff is more cooperative. I find myself examining my behaviors and the significance of the others' behaviors. I'm more aware of the expression of feelings and use it as a cue. I've learned to be more appreciative of others.*
>
> *We feel good about ourselves. The role of our facilitator helped. You made us feel respected. We felt that you were here for our needs, to help us express ourselves freely and determine our own agenda. You often took a back seat, allowing us to interact. You showed openness, receptivity, and acceptance. Your sharing of stories was very helpful. They let us know that you had "been there," that you recognize that what we do is difficult. We knew that we had time for ourselves, time to think. It made us feel important, that we count.*

Positive changes resulting from a caring action are based on the criterion of the welfare for whom the caring action is carried out (Gaut, 1983, 1986). The criterion of the head nurses' welfare was therefore deemed to be met.

While exploring the caring components of nursing, the head nurses seemed to come naturally to an awareness that they could promote the caring of patients by demonstrating caring of their personnel. Our discussions were consistent with the theories of caring and with proposals promoting the integration of these theories into nursing administration practice. I, therefore, evaluated as satisfactory the relationship between the discussion and the reference framework provided, fulfilling provisions of the second criterion.

TOWARDS A THEORETICAL STATEMENT

From the foregoing experience, it appears that caring can enrich nursing managers' reflective thinking and be useful in helping head nurses to develop and to grow within the working environment. Accountable managers create an environment which enables others to fulfill themselves and, therefore, offer high quality nursing care. In addition, nurse managers are entrusted with the responsibility of articulating values, meanings, and the essential attributes of nursing so that our professional service is seen as highly valuable and caring an integral part of nursing care.

According to those authors who discuss caring in relation to nursing administration (Dunham, 1989; Jennings, 1987; Miller, 1987; Nyberg, 1990), the underlying philosophy of current management theories is grounded in an empirical or traditional scientific worldview, which paradigm is based on beliefs in absolutes, in objectivity, and in the autonomous independent order of facts and principles regardless of their historical or sociocultural context. A bureaucratic value system of cost-efficiency, productivity, predictability, reliability, control, high technology, and political competition promotes allegiance to the institution. Its structures maintain subordination and uniformity. The products of goods and commodities are regulated by materials, skills, and speed. The goals of organizational health and survival focus on economic principles and generally avoid humanistic values. As a result, human welfare may suffer in the institutional environment with efficiency diminishing as individuals are devalued.

Providing an important contrast, and as a philosophical under-pinning of nursing, is the perceived holistic view or historicism (Dunham, 1989; Jennings, 1987; Miller, 1987; Nyberg, 1989). This human science paradigm includes beliefs that the actions of humans are free willed, that truth and facts are dynamic and subjective and occur within the natural phenomena which emerge from the inter-actions between persons and environments. It is the professional value system that fosters allegiance to patients, society, and the profession. Value is given to subjectivity, kindness, moral concern, respect, personal autonomy, authority, responsibility, accountability, self-actualization, and optimal human functioning within participative management modes. Products of positive changes in health status, personal well being, and human survival, eclectic and holistic in nature, are evaluated by behavioral processes from diverse knowledge bases.

In this project, a facilitating group experience enabled head nurses to articulate caring, increase their awareness of its meaning to one another, and enhance caring in practice. From this experience, a tentative theoretical statement rises: As caring is advocated by a facilitative nursing leader within a small group experience, nurses who benefit from the experience will exhibit caring behaviors toward their patients and peers, and will interact in a healthy way within the organizational context.

As one head nurse exclaimed:

> What I learned here really works! I just helped a nurse to truly care for a family. If the incident had happened before we started meeting together I would have handled things very differently. I wouldn't even have seen what was really going on.

The preceding description of a strategy to promote caring is some-what limited for those who might wish to repeat the experience. Therefore, a brief summary follows. Based on Gaut's action descrip-tion of caring, the need for caring enhancement within the organiza-tional culture of an acute care hospital was established (Gaut, 1983, 1986; Leininger, 1980, 1988a,b,d; Ray, 1987, 1988a,b, 1989). The goal was to enable head nurses to integrate caring behaviors into their daily activities (Gaut, 1983, 1986). As the experience of being cared for affects the ability to care (Roach, 1984, 1987), the chosen tactic was to exhibit caring behaviors toward nurse managers through facilitative leadership (Gaut, 1983, 1986; Watson, 1985a, 1985b). The tactic, implemented within the context of a group experience favoured dynamic reciprocal transpersonal relationships among participants (Gaut, 1983, 1986; Watson, 1985a,b). The outcome, positive change, was based on the criterion of the welfare of the head nurses for whom the action was intended (Gaut, 1983, 1986) and on the integration of caring into their practice.

It would seem that this outline of a strategy to promote caring, as it evolved, is an appropriate means by which the caring components of clinical and administrative nursing can be explored. This participative research study assisted in the blending of caring knowledge with administrative activities and the identification of factors necessary to the promotion of caring within the particular context. The subsequent clarification of the dimensions of the head nurse's role permitted the adoption of caring approaches by them towards each other and their staff. This initiated a rapprochement of clinical and administrative nurses, lessening the feelings of solitude of the latter. The content of the discussions closely resembles the five attributes of a caring nursing administrator identified by Nyberg (1989): commitment, self-worth, ability to set priorities, openness, and ability to bring out potential. It also could be said that the apparent integration of caring knowledge was conducive to the creation of a climate of support on the unit (Jennings, 1987).

REFERENCES

Barrett-Lennard, G. T. (1975). Process, effects and structure in intensive groups: A theoretical descriptive analysis. In C. L. Cooper (Ed.), *Theories of group processes*. Toronto: John Wiley & Sons, 59–86.

Baumgart, A., & Larsen, J. (1988). Overview: Inside nursing workplaces. In A. Baumgart & J. Larsen (Eds.), *Canadian nursing faces the future. Development and change*. Toronto: C.V. Mosby, 179–189.

Benner, P., & Wrubel, J. (1989). *The primacy of caring: Stress and coping in health and illness*. Menlo Park, CA: Addison-Wesley.

Blair, E. (1989). Nursing and administration: A synthesis model. *Nursing Administration Quarterly, 13*(2), 1–11.

Chaska, V. L. (1983). Theories of nursing and organizations: Generating integrated models for administration practice. In L. Chaska (Ed.), *The nursing profession. A time to speak.* New York: McGraw-Hill, 720–731.

Christenson, P. J. (1988). An ethical framework for nursing service administration. *Advances in Nursing Science, 10*(3), 46–55.

Claus, K. E., & Bailey, J. T. (1977). *Power and influence in health care: A new approach to leadership.* St. Louis: C.V. Mosby.

Culbert, S. A. (1975). Conscious raising: A five-stage model for social and organizational change. In C.L. Cooper (Ed.), *Theories of group processes.* Toronto: John Wiley & Sons, 87–102.

Dunham, J. (1989). The art of humanistic nursing administration: Expanding the horizons. *Nursing Administration Quarterly, 13*(3), 55–66.

Gaut, D. A. (1983). Development of a theoretically adequate description of caring. *Western Journal of Nursing Research, 5*(4), 312–324.

Gaut, D. A. (1986). Evaluating caring competencies in nursing practice. *Topics in Clinical Nursing, 8*(2), 77–83.

Gaut, D. A. (1988). A theoretical description of caring as action. In M. Leininger (Ed.), *Care: The essence of nursing and health.* Detroit: Wayne State University, 27–44.

Gaylin, W. (1976). *Caring.* New York: Avon.

Harris, P. L. (1984). Burnout in nursing administration. *Nursing Administration Quarterly, 8*(3), 61–70.

Harris, R. (1989). Reviewing nursing stress according to a proposed coping-adaption framework. *Advances in Nursing Science, 11*(2), 12–18.

Hillestad, E. (1984). Is it lonely at the top? *Nursing Administration Quarterly, 8*(3), 1–13.

Hogue, J.-P., Levesque, D., & Morin, E. M. (1988). *Groupe, pouvoir et communication.* Québec: Université du Québec.

Jennings, B. M. (1987). Social support: A way to a climate of caring. *Nursing Administration Quarterly, 11*(4), 63–71.

Jennings, B. M., & Meleis, A. I. (1988). Nursing theory and administrative practice: Agenda for the 1990's. *Advances in Nursing Science, 10*(3), 56–69.

Lakin, M., & Costanzo, P. R. (1975). The leader and the experiential group. In C. L. Cooper (Ed.), *Theories of group processes.* Toronto: John Wiley & Sons, 205–234.

Leininger, M. M. (1980, October). "Caring" a central focus of nursing and health care services. *Nursing and Health Care,* 135–142.

Leininger, M. M. (1985). Ethnography and ethnonursing: Models and modes of qualitative data analysis. In M. M. Leininger (Ed.), *Qualitative research methods in nursing*. Orlando, FL: Grune & Stratton, 33–73.

Leininger, M. M. (1988a). The phenomenon of caring: Importance, research questions and theoretical considerations. In M. M. Leininger (Ed.), *Caring: An essential human need*. Detroit: Wayne State University, 3–15.

Leininger, M. M. (1988b). Care: The essence of nursing and health. In M. M. Leininger (Ed.), *Care: The essence of nursing and health*. Detroit: Wayne State University, 3–15.

Leininger, M. M. (1988c). Caring is nursing: Understanding the meaning, importance, and issues. In M. M. Leininger (Ed.), *Care: The essence of nursing and health*. Detroit: Wayne State University, 83–93.

Leininger, M. M. (1988d). History, issues, and trends in the discovery and uses of care in nursing. In M. M. Leininger (Ed.), *Care: Discovery and uses in clinical and community nursing*. Detroit: Wayne State University, 1–26.

Lieberman, M. A., Yalom, I. D., & Miles, M. B. (1973). *Encounter groups: First Facts*. New York: Basic Books.

Marz, N. S. (1986). Conceptual care model for reducing stress of newly employed nurses (summary). The care symposium. Considerations for nurse administrators. *The Journal of Nursing Administration, 16*(1), 25–30.

Mayeroff, M. (1971). *On caring*. New York: Harper & Row.

Miller, K. L. (1987). The human care perspective in nursing administration. *The Journal of Nursing Administration, 17*(2), 10–12.

Nyberg, J. (1989). The element of caring in nursing administration. *Nursing Administration Quarterly, 13*(3), 9–16.

Nyberg, J. (1990). Human care and economics: Foundations of nursing administration practice. *Advances in Nursing Science, 13*(1), 74–78.

Order of Nurses of Québec. (1989). *Hypertension: L'urgence des choix*. Author.

Québec Hospital Association. (1988). *L'infirmière, force vive du centre hospitalier* (Mémoire). Montréal: Q.H.A.: Direction des communications.

Ray, M. A. (1987). Technological caring: A new model in critical care. *Dimensions of Critical Care Nursing, 6*(3), 166–173.

Ray, M. A. (1988a). A philosophical analysis of caring within nursing. In M. M. Leininger, *Caring: An essential human need*. Detroit: Wayne State University, 25–35.

Ray, M. A. (1988b). The development of a classification system of institutional caring. In M. M. Leininger, Care: The essence of nursing and health. Detroit: Wayne State University, 95–112.

Ray, M. A. (1989). The theory of bureaucratic caring for nursing practice in the organizational culture. Nursing Administration Quarterly, 13(2), 31–42.

Roach, M. S. (1984). The human mode of being. Implications for nursing. (Perspectives in Caring. Monograph No. 1). Toronto: University of Toronto, Faculty of Nursing.

Roach, M. S. (1987). The human act of caring: A blueprint for the health profession. Ottawa: Canadian Hospital Association.

Rogers, C. R. (1970). Carl Rogers on encounter groups. New York: Harper & Row.

Rowland, H., & Rowland, B. (1985). Nursing administration handbook (2nd ed.). Rockville, MD: Aspen.

Scalzi, C. (1988). Role stress and coping strategies of nurse executives. Journal of Nursing Administration, 18(3), 34–38.

Schutz, W. C. (1966). The Interpersonal underworld. A reprint edition of FIRO-A three-dimensional theory of interpersonal behaviour. Palo Alto, CA: Science & Behaviour Book.

Stevens, B. J. (1983). Applying nursing theory in nursing administration. In L. Chaska (Ed.) The nursing profession: A time to speak. New York: McGraw-Hill, 708–719.

Stevens, B. J. (1985). The nurse as an executive (3rd ed.). Rockville, MD: Aspen.

Watson, J. (1985a). Nursing: The philosophy and science of caring (2nd ed.). Boulder, CO: Associated University Press.

Watson, J. (1985b). Nursing: Human science and human care. East Norwalk, CT: Appleton-Century-Crofts.

Watson, J. (1988, August). New dimensions of human care theory. Nursing Science Quarterly, 175–181.

Yalom, I. D. (1985). The theory and practice of group psychotherapy (3rd ed.). New York: Basic Books.

7

Evaluation Research within the Human Caring Framework

Ruth M. Neil
Carole A. Schroeder

Evaluation is an investment in people and in progress." These words succinctly express the values inherent in Lincoln and Guba's (1989) *Fourth Generation Evaluation* and are shared by the authors of this paper. Lincoln and Guba identified the following seven characteristics of evaluation which are consistent with human caring values:

1. Social, cultural, and political factors need to be viewed as integral and meaningful components of the evaluation process.
2. Evaluation is a joint, collaborative process that aims at the evolution of consensual constructions about that which is being evaluated.
3. Evaluation is a teaching/learning process in which all stakeholders are both teachers and learners.

4. Evaluation is a continuous, recursive, and highly divergent process. All reconstructions that emerge from an evaluation are considered not as "truth," but as the most informed and sophisticated constructions that are possible at this time.

5. Evaluation is an emergent process. While the process is going on, as new information emerges, the evaluator is duty-bound to follow wherever it leads.

6. Evaluation is a process with unpredictable outcomes.

7. Evaluation is a process that creates reality. The term "findings" suggests the presence of objective truths and does not take into account the human values and interpersonal negotiations which occur during the evaluation process.

PURPOSES

This paper has two purposes. The first is to acquaint readers with the Denver Nursing Project in Human Caring (DNPHC or the Caring Center). The second is to describe two projects which each provided valuable evaluation information concerning the experiences of clients at DNPHC.

One of the projects—the use of focus groups—was designed specifically for the purpose of program evaluation. The processes involved in using focus groups are very consistent with the characteristics described by Lincoln and Guba (1985). The other project—the production of a videotape about the Caring Center—was planned to accomplish other goals, but emerged as an evaluative document very relevant to the Center's mission and objectives.

It is not the authors' intent to provide an in-depth discussion of advantages/disadvantages of either method, or to establish an argument favoring one over the other. Rather, we wish to share our reflective thoughts on why both approaches are appropriate in the human caring framework.

THE DENVER NURSING PROJECT IN HUMAN CARING

The Denver Nursing Project in Human Caring is a nurse-directed outpatient facility serving persons with HIV/AIDS. DNPHC has been open since July, 1988, and, to date, has recorded more than 8,000 client visits. Sponsorship of the Center is shared by a grant from the Department of Health and Human Services (which began in July, 1990), the University of Colorado School of Nursing, and three Denver hospitals. Persons eligible to participate in services of the center are those who obtain their primary HIV care through one of the participating hospitals.

At the Center, clients participate in outpatient medical treatments and numerous nurse-designed supportive programs which include, but are not limited to, intravenous fluids, blood transfusions, Pentamidine treatments, nutrition assistance (complimentary meals as well as nutrition information), massage, therapeutic touch, support groups, stress management classes including aerobics, peer support, opportunity for volunteer and paid services to the center, and referrals to other agencies. In addition to client services, the Center has missions related to education and research.

Based on Jean Watson's theory of human care nursing, the Mission Statement of DNPHC expresses respect for the uniqueness and individuality of each person and belief that health and well-being are multidimensional. Also expressed is the belief that each person has the right and responsibility to make informed choices concerning life values and health, and that individual healing processes can be strengthened through authentic caring relationships.

The commitment to individuality in defining health and personal values and to the importance of caring relationships provided the basis for choice of evaluation methods described here. The meaning and success of any given experience a client has at the center must be defined by that client. Thus, the evaluation method needs to provide opportunity for clients to express their experiences in personal terms. As Watson wrote, "We can choose to study the inner world of experiences rather than the outer world of observation. We can choose to be a part of our method and involved in the clinical research process rather than be distant, objectively remote, and primarily concerned with the product of science" (Bevis & Watson, 1988, p. 274).

FOCUS GROUP METHODOLOGY

During the fall of 1990, focus group methodology was chosen to evaluate the programs and services of DNPHC. Focus groups are an inductive method of qualitative research used to obtain information from the participants' point of view rather than the researchers' view. As discussed by Des Rosier and Zellers (1989), focus groups provide a forum for innovative solutions to chronic problems and a process whereby groups can visualize and define the complexity of problems and solutions (p. 21). Focus groups are conducted in a natural environment in which participants mutually influence each other while the moderator facilitates and focuses discussion by listening, observing, and collecting the information (Kreuger, 1988).

From a research perspective, advantages of the method include low cost, social orientation, natural setting, dynamics of group interaction, group ownership of problems and solutions, speed of results, sample size, and high face validity (Kreuger, 1988). Many of these characteristics are particularly relevant for the population of DNPHC. Due to the progressive and debilitating nature of HIV infection, in a caring framework, priority must be given to responsiveness to continually changing needs of clients, in order to offer appropriate assistance. Krueger listed the common tendency to implement results before evaluating all sources of information (because of the high face validity of clients' stories) as a possible disadvantage of this method. When serving people who "don't have a lot of time," however, this tendency may *not* be disadvantageous.

USING THE PROCESS

At DNPHC, a total of 51 participants took part in a total of eight focus group sessions. There were five client groups, basically identified as follows: (1) persons with a long-term history of HIV disease, (2) acutely ill persons, (3) newly diagnosed or new to the center, (4) women, and (5) family, friends, and lovers. The other three groups were comprised of the staffs of the infectious disease clinics of the three sponsoring hospitals.

Moderators for the focus group sessions were persons knowledgeable about the goals and programs of DNPHC and who had experience in group dynamics. As is recommended in focus group literature, the moderators were not regular care providers or administrative staff of the Center. Sessions lasted approximately one and one-half hours each. Recording was accomplished by the presence of two note takers. The facilitators used a flip chart to make visible to the group the major concerns and themes that emerged.

To fulfill the ideal that focus groups are concerned with the participants' point of view, rather than the researchers', the format for each session consisted of only two requests from the moderator:

1. We are interested in people sharing their ideas and opinions on the Center's operations. Please think back to what the Center does well, and we'll talk about how these things can be developed.
2. Please think back to what could be improved about the Center's operations and give us some ideas on this subject.

Data analysis consisted of a general qualitative descriptive method, based on Lincoln and Guba (1985) and Field and Morse (1986). Information was considered from the perspective of its commonality across groups as well as how perceptions varied from group to group.

A summary of responses which endorsed the Center included:

Caring behaviors

Support groups/peer support

Treatments

Nonclinical environment

Education/information

A summary of responses which indicated areas for improvement included:

Hours (need to be expanded)

Emergency phone support program

Specialized support groups

Group facilitator methodology

Vary meeting times for support groups

Suggestions for educational offerings

Follow-up/orientation of new clients

Improve social services/financial counselling

Continuity of staff

Publicity

Parking/transportation

The focus group methodology proved itself to be a humanistic means of evaluating consumer satisfaction congruent with Watson's theory of human caring. Different concerns of clients in different stages of the disease process were elicited by the clients telling their stories about living with AIDS. The stories were both moving and informative to the researchers and also provided the opportunity for clients to share their frustrations with one another and with the group moderators and note-takers. Recently, Sandelowski (1991) pointed out that "informants . . . by virtue of being human . . . are already engaged in the very human act of story-telling" (p. 164). The authors believe that an important aspect of human caring is allowing and encouraging people to tell their stories. Clients experienced feeling valued and cared for in exchange for the information being imparted.

After reviewing the themes that emerged during the focus group discussion, the Center staff increased the number of hours per week the facility is open, carefully considered emergency telephone support options, and offered "specialized" support groups (e.g., a women's group and psychoeducation on topics such as managing anger and substance abuse). Focus groups will continue to be used periodically at DNPHC, in addition to other methods, for ongoing evaluation of our efforts to be authentically caring in our relationships with those we serve.

THE VIDEOTAPE EXPERIENCE

In the spring of 1990, DNPHC received a grant from the Aetna Life Insurance Company for the purpose of producing a videotape "to tell the Center story." The objectives for the project included having a resource to use for client recruitment and for education. Because of the process used to produce the tape, it inadvertently became an evaluative document in its own right.

The staff members who had written the grant request invited participation from clients, center staff, and volunteers in "brainstorming" about what should be taped. A videographer who was very interested in the mission and programs of DNPHC was hired to organize a "shooting schedule." In a sense, he became the qualitative researcher. He was involved in a human as well as in a technical manner during the entire filming process. Collier and Collier (1986) pointed out that ". . . only human response can open the camera's eye to its meaningful use in research" (p. 5).

Information about borrowing the videotape, "It's Nice to Be Loved" can be obtained from the authors at the following address: Denver Nursing Project in Human Caring, DVAMC Building #5, 1055 Clermont Street, Denver, CO 80220.

Various staff members and clients were invited to be interviewed on camera and respond to open-ended questions about what the Center meant to them. As footage accumulated and was reviewed, a few "more directive" questions were added to assure that all the major programs and services of DNPHC were included. Finally, minimal pre-planning of one scene was done to provide the phrase which became the title for the finished document—"It's Nice to Be Loved."

The videographer and staff members in charge of the project edited and sequenced what can best be described as a collage of staff and client "testimonials" about the meaning and value in their own lives of caring relationships at DNPHC. Short vignettes from these interviews include the following:

"If I could stay overnight, I would."

"This is more like a home to me than any place I've ever been."

"The staff is concerned about every aspect of the clients' lives, not just the physical."

"What there's more of here than anything else is lots of love."

"It's like having a hospital in your home."

PROCESS AND PRODUCT

A positive addendum to the videotape experience, similar to the focus group methodology, was the probable therapeutic value of the process. During the ten weeks that the videotape was being filmed, it was common to overhear clients asking other clients or staff, "Have you been taped yet? How do you think you did? I hope it comes out 'good'. It was nice to be included." When the tape was finished, the activity room at the Center was full of interested, proud "new stars." The sense of shared accomplishment felt among staff and clients carried forward into several other projects in the months that followed.

CONCLUSION

Both the focus group methodology and the production of the videotape allowed clients and staff of the Denver Nursing Project in Human Caring to experience the realization of the evaluation characteristics Lincoln and Guba (1989) listed as being consistent with human caring values. Our continuing commitment to the evolving nature of each person helps us to believe that, like with life in general, evaluative processes are unpredictable and do create reality.

REFERENCES

Bevis, E. O., & Watson, J. (1988). *Toward a caring curriculum: A new pedagogy for nursing.* New York: National League for Nursing.

Collier, J., & Collier, M. (1986). *Visual anthropology: Photography as a research method.* Albuquerque, NM: University of New Mexico Press.

Des Rosier, M., & Zellers, K. (1989). Focus groups: A program planning technique. *Journal of Nursing Administration, 19*(3), 20–25.

Field, P., & Morse, J. (1985). *Nursing research: The application of qualitative approaches.* Rockville, MD: Aspen Publications.

Guba, E. G., & Lincoln, Y. S. (1989). *Fourth generation evaluation.* Newbury Park, CA: SAGE.

Kreuger, R. (1988). *Focus groups.* Beverly Hills: Sage.

Lincoln, Y., & Guba, E. (1985). *Naturalistic inquiry.* London: Sage.

Sandelowski, M. (1991). Telling stories: Narrative approaches in qualitative research. *Image 23*(3), 161–166.

8

The Impact of Nurse Caring on Patient Outcomes

Joanne R. Duffy

Nursing and the promotion of health is human-oriented. The human-to-human contact which nurses have with patients in the hospital setting is unlike that of any other health professional. Nurses, while helping patients with activities of daily living, nutrition and elimination patterns, mobility, and knowledge of their illness develop personal relationships with patients and families. According to King (1981), purposeful nurse–patient relationships lead to transactions and ultimately goal attainment. Watson (1979), however, submits that in order to promote growth and personal meaning, the nurse–patient relationship must be of a caring nature.

Caring is a fundamental component of nursing (Henry, 1975) that has been linked to positive patient outcomes by nurse theorists (Henderson, 1964; Leininger, 1981; Orlando, 1961; Travelbee, 1966; Watson, 1985). It consists of values, attitudes, and behaviors that occur within the nurse–patient relationship. Caring is a process composed of both instrumental (physical) acts and expressive (relationship) behaviors (Watson, 1981). Hospitalized patients and families expect nurses to be personal and concerned, as well as skillful technicians (Cohn, 1988).

Despite the fact that caring is considered foundational to nursing, non-caring behaviors in hospitals do exist and account for needless patient and family anxiety (Kelly, 1988). Consider the following example: A 55-year-old male described experiences with hospital nurses as cold, rough, and uncomfortable.

> *Any contact that I had with those nurses down there, you know it was cold and it certainly makes you feel helpless to be strapped on a bed and in such pain and when anyone speaks to you, even the sound of their voice doesn't sound very concerned. One nurse was washing me up, and oh, she was so rough! Just like she was washing a doll and not a human being. I remember the nurse bathing me, and just her movements, they were so rough, very rough physically. You know, she'd run the razor, well almost like striking out at someone. They did not make me feel comfortable or that I was of any value to them. And I suppose all of us like to feel that we're valuable. (Reimen, 1986, p. 30)*

The example portrays a serious problem in today's health care institutions. Kelly (1988) recently discussed her concerns about the lack of human dignity afforded to four elderly patients by professional nurses. Descriptions of the nurses' actions included causing unnecessary pain and treating the patients as incompetent nuisances. All these incidences occurred in well-respected American hospitals. As Kelly (1988) pointed out, "the patients did not expect extra special treatments; they did expect nurses to care or at least act as if they did" (p. 17).

Proudfoot (1983) spoke to nurses as having "hurry sickness." In other words, nurses tend to focus on the many tasks they have to complete so that they appear to hurry from one to the other without any time to spare. Clinical experience supports that patients view this as "no one cares."

Jourard (1971) described the defensive behavior of nurses. He maintained that nurses "wear a coat of armor" in order to avoid the terrible patient situations they encounter. This suit of armor creates the appearance that nurses are cold, indifferent, and unconcerned about patients and families. In fact, Jourard (1971) stated that nurses protect themselves from the realities of the hospital environment by acting this way.

Reports of non-caring nurse behaviors have resulted in patients' feeling uncomfortable, helpless, devalued, painful, and uneasy (Drew, 1986; Kelly, 1988; Reimen, 1986). These feelings are not representative of hospitalized patients' expectations and are contrary to the goals of nursing. It is reasonable to consider, then, that nurse caring may be linked to patient outcomes. Watson's (1985) theory of human care supports this notion and became the theoretical base for this study. Knowledge of the degree of nurse caring and its relationship to patient outcomes will describe nursing's unique contribution to patient care.

PURPOSE

This study measured the relationships between nurse caring behaviors and the selected outcomes of patient satisfaction, health status, length of stay, and nursing care costs in hospitalized medical and/or surgical patients.

REVIEW OF THE LITERATURE

The phenomenon of caring has been studied philosophically (Gaut, 1984; Mayerhoff, 1970), spiritually (Hovde, 1975; Roach, 1987), as a value (Noddings, 1984; Pellegrino, 1985), theoretically (Leininger, 1981; Watson, 1985), ethnographically (Leininger, 1978; 1981; 1984) and in many clinical situations. As a human activity, caring has been associated with full development and survival of the human species throughout the world (Leininger, 1984). According to Mayerhoff (1970), caring is a process through which development occurs both in the recipient and the caregiver. Noddings (1984) views caring as a feminine value, one that comes naturally to women while Pellegrino (1985) asserts that caring is the moral obligation of health professionals.

In her studies of expert nurses, Benner (1984) describes the power associated with caring. She states that "almost no intervention will work if the nurse–patient relationship is not based on mutual trust and genuine caring" (p. 209). She further emphasizes that caring is "what makes expert nurses effective" (Benner & Wrubel, 1989, p. 4).

In clinical studies, patients have identified behaviors that provoke feelings of being cared for by nurses. The meaning of caring has been studied transculturally (Leininger, 1978; 1981), within a home-health population (Henry, 1975), and in hospitalized patients (Brown, 1986). Both instrumental and expressive behaviors have been identified by patients as indicators of nurse caring. In two oncology populations, patients emphatically identified competent clinical skills as indicators of caring (Larson, 1984; Mayer, 1987).

Similar results also were found in a sample of myocardial infarction patients (Cronin & Harrison, 1988). These patients reported physical care and monitoring as most indicative of nurse caring. The life-threatening nature of these diagnostic patient groups support this view.

Conversely, when nurses have been asked to identify the meaning of caring, expressive behaviors are most frequently cited (Ford, 1981; Larson, 1987; Mayer, 1987). In a small sample ($n = 8$) of intensive care unit nurses, Ray (1987) examined caring from the nurses' point of view. The nurses described several dimensions of caring including growth, technical competence, sharing, communication, and decision making. Most believed, however, that technical competence must first be mastered in order for caring to occur.

While theories of caring have evolved (Leininger, 1981; Watson, 1979; 1985) and the meaning of caring has been studied extensively, nothing has been reported regarding the consequences or the impact of nurse caring on patient outcomes.

According to Merry (1987), patient outcomes offer new opportunities to provide decision makers with information that directly translates into economic terms. The linkage of nursing activities and behaviors to patient outcomes may ultimately impact institutional policy, staffing patterns, salaries for nurses, the focus on technology and tasks, and continuing education. Four outcomes that have been linked to nursing's continuous interaction with patients and families during hospitalization are patient satisfaction, health status, length of stay (LOS), and nursing care costs (Abramowitz, Berry, & Cote, 1986;

Hinshaw, Gerber, Atwood, & Allen, 1983; Hinshaw, Scofield, & Atwood, 1981; King, 1981; Marchette & Halloman, 1986; Watson, 1985).

Although satisfaction with hospital services is a subjective opinion from the patients' point of view, it is now recognized as a legitimate outcome of care (Nelson & Goldstein, 1989). Patient satisfaction implies gratification of needs and fulfillment of expectations (Risser, 1975).

Although considerable variability exists in methodology, over 30 years of research on patient satisfaction has yielded three consistent results: (1) in general, patients are usually highly satisfied with hospital services; (2) demographic characteristics do not seem to be a factor in patient satisfaction; and (3) satisfaction with nursing care is a consistent factor in overall satisfaction with hospitalization (Abramowitz, Berry, & Cote, 1986; Cassareal, Mills, & Plant, 1986; Cleary & McNeal, 1988; Miller-Bader, 1988). It is reasonable to expect this last conclusion since nurses are in constant interaction with patients. For example, in a study of eight hospitals, nursing staff accounted for the strongest factor in overall satisfaction (Cassareal et al., 1986). This finding is consistent with the views of Abramowitz, Berry, and Cote who found that positive interactions with nurses was the strongest predictor of overall patient satisfaction. Similarly, Feinholtz (1986) asked patients in Los Angeles to rank 30 factors that they considered important satisfiers. "Respondents repeatedly stated that they wanted demonstrated attention and communication . . . they would like to be treated like human beings and ones whose time is valuable . . . the consumer's primary concern is how he/she is treated as a person" (p. 79). These are aspects of care that have traditionally involved nursing but which have not been specifically examined with regard to patient satisfaction.

Regaining health, another important outcome variable (Donabedian, 1980; King, 1981) is foremost in patients' minds (Kanar, 1988) during hospitalization. According to Donabedian, a level of health that allows one to perform activities of daily living (ADLs) is sought after in this country and is a goal of hospitalization. Of course, promoting health and improving health status is the goal of nursing (King, 1981).

Becker and Naiman (1980) maintain that "nurses, by virtue of their numbers and patient contact, have the greatest potential of any group of health professionals for exerting an impact on patients health behaviors" (p. 130). Unfortunately, no research has been found regarding the impact of nurses' human caring behaviors on the health status of patients while hospitalized.

The length of time a patient spends in a hospital is directly related to the cost of providing care (Halloran, 1983). With the advent of prospective payment, nursing and hospital administrators are being forced to examine length of stay as reimbursement rates are tied to this outcome measure. From the patients' view, time spent in the hospital is time spent away from family, friends, and work. Although this personal cost is difficult to measure, it is very real. According to Davis-Martin (1986), the success of a hospital in the prospective payment system is directly related to LOS.

Sustained contact with nurses supports prevention and early detection of complications (Munson et al., 1980) which may affect LOS. The impact of the human interacting aspect of nursing on LOS, however, has not been reported.

Not only do today's health care consumers expect satisfactory service and renewed health status in a shorter period of time, they are concerned about the cost of this service. Costs imply value or equity and represent the use of resources. As such, their measurement assesses the efficiency of an operation (Hassenein, 1987) and represents still another important patient outcome variable (Donabedian, 1980). Costs for hospital services is a concern not only of patients and the federal government (HCFA, 1989), but also of nursing administrators (Schaffer, 1987) since costs for nursing care contribute a sizeable component of the total cost of hospital care (Walker, 1983).

It is reasonable to consider that nurses, who frequently interact with patients and families, have an influence on the costs for hospital services. Commonly, studies examining nursing costs are associated with nursing care delivery systems, staffing patterns, and the use of nurse practitioners (Kamaroff, Sawayer, Flatley, & Brown, 1976; Hinshaw, Scofield, & Atwood, 1981; Lewis, Resnick, Schmidt, & Waxman, 1969; Scott, Forrest, & Brown, 1976). The impact of the human nurse–patient interaction process on nursing care costs has not been reported.

In summary, professional nurses, a large component of the health care system with whom patients frequently interact, have a logical influence on the effectiveness and efficiency of that system. The impact of the daily human contact between patient and nurse on patient outcomes has not been reported.

ASSUMPTIONS

1. The essence of nursing is caring (Leininger, 1981).
2. Although they may be viewed differently, favorable patient outcomes are valued by nurses and patients.
3. The respondents responded truthfully to all questionnaires.
4. Caring can be measured.

RESEARCH HYPOTHESES

H1 There will be a positive relationship between nurse caring behaviors and patient satisfaction in hospitalized medical and/or surgical patients.

H2 There will be a positive relationship between nurse caring behaviors and perception of health status in hospitalized medical and/or surgical patients.

H3 There will be an inverse relationship between nurse caring behaviors and LOS in hospitalized medical and/or surgical patients.

H4 There will be an inverse relationship between nurse caring behaviors and nursing care costs in hospitalized medical and/or surgical patients.

METHODS

The author selected a descriptive correlational research design to investigate the study hypotheses. In addition, the author selected a quantitative approach to identify significant relationships between the independent variable, nurse caring behaviors, and the dependent variables of patient satisfaction, health status, LOS, and nursing care costs. The setting for the study was a voluntary, 500-bed university teaching hospital in a large metropolitan area of the eastern United States serving mainly an urban and suburban population.

Sample

The author selected a purposive, random sample of 86 subjects based on the following criteria: (1) medical and/or surgical diagnosis; (2) age 21 years or greater; (3) hospitalized at least 48 hours; (4) ability to understand the English language; and (5) displayed no confusion and/or critical illness. The sample size was based on a medium effect, an alpha level of .05 and a power of 80 percent (Cohen & Cohen, 1975). In total, the author selected and approached 99 subjects with 86 subjects actually agreeing to participate.

Instrumentation

The five instruments used to collect the data for this study are as follows: (1) the Caring Assessment Tool (CAT), designed by the researcher, was used to measure nurse caring; (2) the Patient Satisfaction Visual Analog Scale (Oberst, 1984) was used as a measure of patient satisfaction; (3) the Sickness Impact Profile (Bergner et al., 1976) measured health status; (4) the Medicus Patient Classification Tool (Medicus, 1975) was used to measure required hours of nursing care per day; and (5) the Patient Information Form, also designed by the researcher, collected demographic and descriptive data.

The Caring Assessment Tool was designed to meet the study purposes and to establish a theoretically based and reliable instrument for use in a diverse patient population (see Figure 1). It consists of 100 items scored in Likert format from 1 (low-caring) to 5 (high-caring) with a possible range of 100 to 500. Psychometric properties of the CAT have been reported elsewhere (Duffy, 1990).

Figure 1
Patient Survey CAT©*

Code No. _____ (1–4)

Card No. _____ (5)

Directions: All of the statements in this survey refer to nursing activities that occur in a hospital. There are five possible responses to each item. They are:

1 = Never
2 = Rarely
3 = Occasionally
4 = Frequently
5 = Always

For each statement, please circle how often you think each activity is occurring during your hospitalization.

Since I have been a patient here, the nurses:

1. Listen to me.   (6)
   1   2   3   4   5

2. Accept me as I am.   (7)
   1   2   3   4   5

3. Treat me kindly.   (8)
   1   2   3   4   5

4. Ignore me.   (9)
   1   2   3   4   5

5. Answer my questions.   (10)
   1   2   3   4   5

6. Include me in their discussions.   (11)
   1   2   3   4   5

7. Respect me.   (12)
   1   2   3   4   5

8. Are more interested in their own problems.   (13)
   1   2   3   4   5

9. Pay attention to me.   (14)
   1   2   3   4   5

10. Enjoy taking care of me.   (15)
    1   2   3   4   5

* © Joanne R. Duffy, R.N., D.N.Sc., (1990), Georgetown University School of Nursing, Washington, D.C.

The Patient Satisfaction Visual Analog Scale (Oberst, 1984) is a one item, horizontal 100 mm line. Scores are derived by measuring in millimeters from left (low satisfaction) to right (high satisfaction) with a possible range of 1 to 100. This visual analogue scale was chosen for its ease and for the reported difficulties in prior measures of patient satisfaction.

The Sickness Impact Profile (SIP) was used to measure perception of health status and is comprised of 189 behavioral items that include activities involved in carrying out one's life. Each item is assigned a weight or scale value indicating its relative severity of dysfunction. Content validity and test-retest reliability studies conducted within 24 hours of each other have been established (Bergner, et al., 1976).

The Medicus Patient Classification Tool was developed in 1975 as a measure of required nursing hours per patient day, an acuity measure. This acuity measure multiplied by the average RN hourly salary and the patient's total LOS became the measure of nursing care costs.

The Patient Information Form was developed by the researcher to collect sample descriptive demographic data. It consists of 11 items such as age, diagnosis, education, etc.

Procedure

Following approval of the research protocol by the institutional review board of the University and the Nursing Research committee, data collection was initiated. This portion of the study extended over a nine-month period from February to October 1989. The computerized midnight census sheet was reviewed for identification of all medical and/or surgical patients. Each patient was assigned a number beginning with 001 and, from this list, a Table of Random Numbers was used to select study participants. Each selected patient was approached to evaluate his or her eligibility based on the sample criteria. The researcher reviewed the informed consent form, obtained the participants' signature and then administered the instruments. All study instruments were completed within 24 hours. To respect confidentiality, the recorded responses were coded and placed in sealed envelopes.

RESULTS

Characteristics of the Study Sample

Of the 86 randomly selected medical and/or surgical patients in this study, the distribution of males (47%) and females (52.3%) was fairly equal. The mean age was 51.3 years. Almost one-half (47.7%) of the study subjects ($n = 41$) were employed full time while 30.2% ($n = 26$) were retired. The mean hospital length of stay at the time of study participation was 11.2 days with a range of 2 to 87 days. For diagnostic categories, acuity levels, hospital days, and other demographic background data, see Table 1.

Description of Major Study Variables

The distribution of scores achieved by hospitalized medical and/or surgical patients on their perceptions of nurse caring behaviors is presented in Table 2. The overall mean score reflects that patients' perceptions of nurse caring was negatively skewed, or hovered toward the higher end of the scale. No studies have been reported which describe this phenomenon of high levels of nurse caring, yet, it is compatible with the inherent actions of nurses as well as nursing theory (Leininger, 1981; Watson, 1979; 1985).

The distribution of patient satisfaction scores revealed a mean of 74.37, also negatively skewed. The location of this distribution is similar to other study samples in that hospitalized patients are generally highly satisfied with their care (Abramowitz, Berry, & Cote, 1986; Cassareal, Mills, & Plant, 1986; Cleary & McNeal, 1988; Miller-Bader, 1988).

Perception of health status scores was relatively low ($m = 18.38\%$). This sample perceived themselves to be rather healthy which is consistent with the acuity data previously cited.

The total LOS and nursing care costs are depicted in Figures 2 and 3. These data are indicative of recent trends in shorter lengths of stay and overall costs for direct nursing care.

Table 1
Demographic Data

		%
Diagnosis	(n = 86)	
Cardiovascular disease		13.0
Diabetes		3.5
Respiratory disease		8.1
Cancer		8.1
Traumatic injury		8.1
Kidney disease		2.3
Surgical operation		36.0
Other		19.8
Acuity	(n = 86)	
Type I		43.0
Type II		36.0
Type III		20.9
Marital Status	(n = 86)	
Married		41.9
Single		30.2
Widower		12.8
Divorced/separated		15.2
Educational Background	(n = 86)	
High School incomplete		15.1
High School graduate		23.3
Some college		15.1
College graduate		16.3
Graduate education		8.1
Post graduate education		14.0
Income Ranges	(n = 86)	
< 15,000/year		18.6
16,000–30,000		40.7
31,000–50,000		23.3
> 50,000		14.0
Missing		3.5

Table 2
Range, Mean, and Standard Deviation of Nurse Caring Behaviors as Perceived by Hospitalized Medical and/or Surgical Patients

	Range (low-high)	M	SD	N
Perceptions of Nurse Caring Behaviors	263–491	387.28	50.55	86

Note. *Interpretation of CAT Score:* 100 = minimum score, nurses never demonstrate caring behaviors as perceived by hospitalized medical and/or surgical patients; 500 = maximum score, nurses always demonstrate caring behaviors as perceived by hospitalized medical and/or surgical patients.

Study Hypotheses

Hypothesis I suggests a positive relationship between nurse caring behaviors and patient satisfaction. A Pearson correlation coefficient revealed a significantly positive relationship between these two variables ($r = .4627$, $p < .001$). To further explore this relationship while controlling for the confounding variables of patient age, acuity, and period of hospitalization, a stepwise multiple regression analysis was performed (see Table 3). None of the confounding variables significantly explained any of the variance associated with patient satisfaction. However, when perceptions of nurse caring behaviors was entered into the equation, an Rsq change of .1868 and F *Change* (4,80) of 19.5715, $p < .001$ was produced. Approximately 19 percent of the variance of patient satisfaction, then, was explained solely by the variable, nurse caring behaviors. Given the magnitude and significance level of this multiple regression analysis, Hypothesis I was fully supported.

Hypothesis II, the existence of a positive relationship between nurse caring behaviors and perceived health status was not supported. The confounding variables of patient acuity and period of hospitalization however, explained close to 16 percent of the variance in perceived health status.

Hypotheses III and IV, the existence of inverse relationships between nurse caring behaviors and total length of stay and nursing

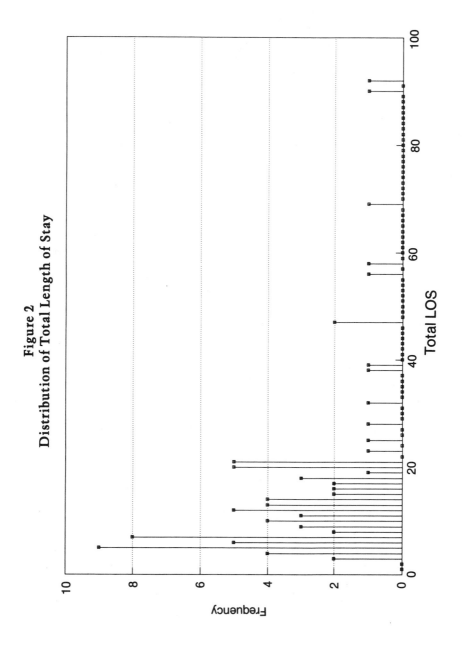

Figure 2
Distribution of Total Length of Stay

126

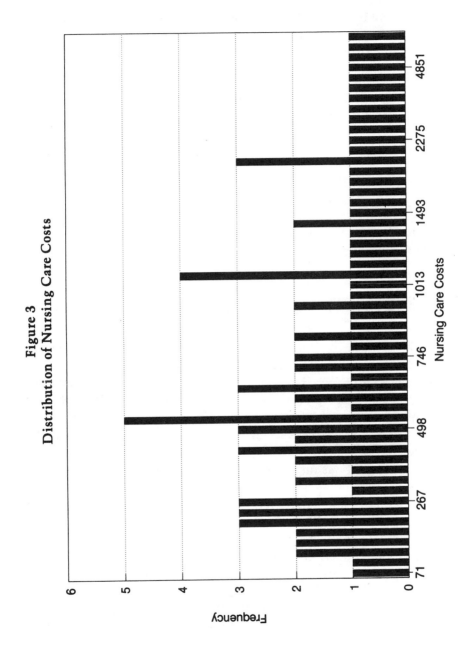

Figure 3
Distribution of Nursing Care Costs

Table 3
Stepwise Multiple Regression of Hospitalized Medical and/or Surgical Patients' Age, Acuity, Period of Hospitalization, and Perceived Nurse Caring Behaviors on Patient Satisfaction.

Step/Variable	Summary Table					
	R	*Rsg*	*RsgCh*	*BETA*	*df*	*FCh*
1. Acuity	.2230	.0497	.0497	−5.75	3,81	1.413
2. Nurse Caring	.4863	.2365	.1868	.2176	4,80	19.57**

Note. $**p < 001$

care costs respectively were not supported. When nurse caring behaviors were entered into these equations, inverse relationships were noted, however, they were not statistically significant.

DISCUSSION

Using Watson's (1985) theory of human care as the theoretical framework for this study, several relationships between nurse caring behaviors and selected patient outcomes were examined. Nurse caring behaviors, operationalized by the CAT, yielded higher scores as expected. Patients in this sample perceived nurses to be more caring which supports theory and reminds us of the core nature of caring among nurses.

Hypothesis I was supported as expected. This finding confirms the work of others in which nursing was found to be significantly correlated with patient satisfaction (Abramowitz, Berry, & Cote, 1986; Cassareal, Mills, & Plant, 1986; Cleary & McNeal, 1988; and Miller-Bader, 1988). This study, however, specifically identifies the caring behaviors of nurses as related to patient satisfaction which is a new finding. It supports Watson's (1979) proposition that nurse caring produces patient satisfaction. It appears that caring nurses are related to satisfied patients, an important indicator of quality (Donabedian, 1980). The fact that no other variables were correlated with patient satisfaction confirms Miller-Bader's (1988) study and contributes to the notion that nurse caring may be an important predictor of patient satisfaction.

Hypotheses II, III, and IV were not supported. Many explanations are plausible for these findings. First, the measure of health status in this study, the SIP, may not have been sensitive enough for this patient population. More specific measures of health status such as relief of symptoms, compliance, comfort, and/or anxiety may have yielded positive results.

Although the subjects were randomly selected, the data support a skewed, more healthy sample. This fact, along with other factors such as patient demographics, may have influenced the measure of health status. The large surgical group of patients in the sample probably contributed to the shorter length of stay and nursing cost data. Typically, surgical patients require less overall nursing time (Medicus, 1975) and the large proportion of these patients in the sample may have accounted for the lower LOS and nursing costs.

Another explanation for these nonsignificant findings may be that the patient sample was so diverse, representing both medical and surgical diagnoses with chronic and acute disease processes, that variance could not be demonstrated. Diagnostic grouping of subjects may have resulted in significant findings.

Finally, the measure of nursing care costs for this sample was derived from the acuity data generated through the Medicus Patient Classification Tool (Medicus, 1975). Although state of the art with established validity and reliability, the tool was not an updated version. This measure, therefore, may not be an accurate reflection of the current acuity of hospitalized medical-surgical patients. Misrepresentation of patient acuity could have interfered with calculation of nursing care costs and impacted the proposed research hypothesis.

Despite the lack of support for these hypotheses, the BETA weights for the relationships of nurse caring behaviors to LOS and nursing care costs were negative. As nurse caring behaviors increased in this study, LOS and nursing care costs declined. Although not significant, these findings indicate a trend in the direction of the original research hypotheses which should be explored in future research.

IMPLICATIONS FOR NURSING AND FUTURE RESEARCH

As this study suggests, the daily commitment to intervening with people who are acutely ill affects patients' outcomes. It is within the practice setting, then, that nursing implications are greatest. Full use of the carative factors (Watson, 1979) in daily nurse-patient interactions provides a foundation for nursing practice. Use of the carative factors, however, requires a commitment on the part of the hospital nurse. Caring as a process means getting involved; this may contradict the hurried, technology-oriented milieu in today's hospitals. Caring requires the courage to change the hospital environment for the betterment of patients and families. Nursing interventions within this caring context become centered on the unique, holistic nature of patients. Relearning and committing to the altruistic values inherent in nursing and appreciation of individual uniqueness are requisites.

In nursing education, faculty must review their conceptual base and perhaps modify it to fit a more interpersonal human interacting approach. Faculty should role-model the carative factors often through creative, sensitizing activities with students. Requiring students to master the carative factors, similarly to mastering procedural techniques, will reinforce the importance of these practices for students in everyday work life. As nursing faculty become caring role models for students, their relationships will focus more on student learning versus faculty teaching.

Finally, nursing administration must find ways to facilitate caring practices in their staff. According to Norris (1989), a double standard presently exists in hospitals. Nurses are supposed to care; yet nursing administrators "demand loyalty, blame instead of problem-solve, sanction excessively harsh punishments, fail to promote self-esteem, fail to allow time for feelings of grief, anger, or failure, and fail to make allowances for nurses' personal concerns" (p. 548). How can staff nurses care in an uncaring environment? How do they know caring behaviors if they have not experienced them?

The vision for nursing administration is clear. Nurses who supervise other nurses must use the carative factors in their daily practice as well. Identifying and operationalizing a conceptual model for practice that includes the use of the carative factors will aid nursing administrators in developing a culture of caring within institutions.

Nursing administrators must demonstrate respect for their employees, maintain sensitivity, let their emotions show judiciously, promote learning and problem solving, and most importantly, begin to understand the subjective meanings that staff nurses attach to their work. This last function requires a certain "clinical presence," a being there, an understanding of the practical aspects of everyday nursing work life. Too often, nursing administrators are involved in activities that keep them in their offices or at all day meetings. Time spent on the clinical units is rare. A reevaluation of the nursing administrator's time is needed. Being clinically present with nursing staff confirms that what they do is important—it reinforces that patients are our reasons for being. It is a method for role-modeling caring, the core of nursing (Watson, 1979).

Nursing administrators must find ways to include the carative factors as essential aspects of nursing on care plans, within patient classification systems, and on performance evaluations. This will reinforce their importance. Regular measurement of nurse caring as perceived by patients will provide valuable insight in quality assurance studies. Finally, rewarding staff for expert caring practices through monetary or advancement awards establishes a value for caring that will be felt throughout the institution.

The implications for further research as a result of this descriptive study are great. First, replication studies will be needed to further examine and validate the findings of this study. Longitudinal studies aimed at examining changes in relationships between nurse caring behaviors and patient outcomes over time would add to the body of knowledge. Studies which seek to link patient demographics to nurse caring and experimental studies which examine the effects of specific caring modalities on patient outcomes are needed to generate administrative changes and affect institutional policies. Finally, nursing educational and administrative studies which link caring practices to staff and student performance could significantly impact the growing knowledge base of nurse caring.

REFERENCES

Abramowitz, S., Berry, E., & Cote, A. (1986). Analyzing patient satisfaction: A multianalytic approach. *Quarterly Review Bulletin, 12*, 122–130.

Alward, R. R. (1983). Patient classification systems: the ideal vs. reality. *The Journal of Nursing Administration, 13*, 14–19.

Becker, M., & Naiman, L. (1980). Strategies for enhancing patient compliance. *Journal of Community Health, 6*, 113–130.

Benner, P. (1984). *From novice to expert.* Menlo Park, CA: Addison-Wesley.

Benner, P., & Wrubel, J. (1989). *The primacy of caring: Stress and coping in health and illness.* Menlo Park, CA: Addison-Wesley.

Bergner, M., Bobbitt, R., Kressel, S., Pollard, W., Gilson, B., & Morris, J. (1976). The sickness impact profile: Conceptual formulation and methodology for the development of a health status measure. *International Journal of Health Services, 6*, 393–412.

Buerhaus, P. (1986). The economics of caring: Challenges and new opportunities for nursing. *Topics in Clinical Nursing, 8*, 13–21.

Brown, L. (1986). The experience of care: Patient perspectives. *Topics in Clinical Nursing, 8*, 56–62.

Cassareal, K. M., Mills, J. I., & Plant, M. A. (1986). Improving service through patient surveys in a multihospital organization. *Hospital and Health Services Administration, 31*, 41–52.

Cleary, P., & McNeal, B. (1988). Patient satisfaction as an indicator of quality of care. *Inquiry, 25*, 25–36.

Cohen, J., & Cohen, P. (1975). *Applied multiple regression/Correlation analysis for the behavioral sciences.* New York: John Wiley & Sons.

Cohn, V. (1988). Expectations of hospitalized patients. *Washington Post,* October 22.

Cronin, S. N., & Harrison, B. (1988). Importance of nurse caring behaviors as perceived by patient with myocardial infarction. *Heart and Lung, 17*, 374–380.

Davis-Martin, S. (1986). Outcome and accountability: Getting into the consumer dimension. *Nursing Management, 17*, 25–29.

Donabedian, A. (1980). *The Definition of quality and approaches to its measurement.* Ann Arbor, MI: Health Administration Press.

Drew, N. (1986). Exclusion and confirmation: A phenomenology of patients' experiences with caregivers. *Image, 18*, 39–43.

Duffy, J. (1990). *The relationship between nurse caring behaviors and selected outcomes of care in hospitalized medical and/or surgical patients.* Unpublished doctoral dissertation. Washington, DC: Catholic University of America.

Feinholz, L. (1986). Using consumer evaluation of health care quality to identify marketing opportunities. *Health Marketing Quarterly, 3,* 73–81.

Ford, M. (1981). Nurse professionals and the caring process. *Dissertation Abstracts International, 43,* 967B–968B.

Gaut, D. (1984). A theoretic description of caring as action. In M. M. Leininger (Ed.), *Care: The essence of nursing and health.* Thorofare, NJ: Slack.

Halloran, E. (1983). The cost dimension of the national joint practice commission demonstration project. *Nursing and Health Care, 6,* 307–313.

Health Care Financing Administration. (1989, October 1). Medicare program—Prospective payments for medicare impatient hospital services. *Federal Register, 71.*

Helman, C. (1978). *Culture, health and illness.* New York: University College Press.

Henderson, V. (1964). The nature of nursing. *American Journal of Nursing, 64,* 62–68.

Henry, O. (1975). Nurse behaviors perceived by patients as indicators of caring. *Dissertation Abstracts International, 36,* 75–76.

Hinshaw, A. S., Scofield, R., & Atwood, J. (1981). Staff, patient, and cost outcomes of all-registered nurse staffing. *Journal of Nursing Administration, 12,* 30–36.

Hinshaw, A. S., Gerber, R., Atwood, J., & Allen, J. (1983). The use of predictive modeling to test nursing practice outcomes. *Nursing Research, 32,* 35–39.

Hinshaw, A. S., & Oakes, D. (1977). Theoretical model testing: patients', nurses' and physicians' expectations for quality nursing care. *Nursing Forum, 10,* 163–187.

Hovde, C. H. (1975). Life's spiritual support. In E. Brown & E. O. Ellis (Eds.), *The later years.* Acton, MA: Publishing Sciences Group.

Jourard, S. (1971). *The transparent self.* New York: Van Nostrand.

Kalisch, B. (1987). Address delivered at the *Nursing Diagnosis Conference.* Washington, DC, March 20.

Kamaroff, J., Sawayer, M., Flatley, S., & Browne, I. (1976). Nurse practitioners' management of common respiratory and genitourinary infections using protocols. *Nursing Research, 25,* 84–89.

Kanar, R. (1988). The influence of a quality assurance program on patient satisfaction. *Journal of Nursing Quality Assurance, 2,* 36–43.

Kelly, L. (1988). The ethic of caring: Has it been discarded? *Nursing Outlook, 36,* 1.

King, I. (1981). *A theory for nursing: Systems, concepts, and process.* New York: John Wiley & Sons.

Larson, P. (1984). Important nurse caring behaviors perceived by patients with cancer. *Oncology Nursing Forum, 11,* 46–50.

Larson, P. (1987). Comparison of cancer patients' and professional nurses' perceptions of important nurse caring behaviors. *Heart and Lung, 16,* 378–382.

Leininger, M. M. (1978). *Transcultural nursing, concepts, theories, practices.* New York: John Wiley & Sons.

Leininger, M. M. (1981). *Care: An essential human need.* Thorofare, NJ: Slack.

Leininger, M. M. (1984). Caring is nursing: Understanding the meaning, importance, and issues. In M. M. Leininger (Ed). *Care: The essence of nursing and health.* Thorofare, NJ: Slack.

Lewis, C., Resnick, B., Schmidt, G., & Waxman, D. (1969). Activities, events, and outcomes of ambulatory care. *New England Journal of Medicine, 280,* 56–61.

Lindeman, C. & VanAerman, B. (1971). Nursing intervention with the pre-surgical patient—the effects of structured and unstructured pre-operative teaching. *Nursing Research, 20,* 319–332.

MacPhearson, K. (1989). Nursing and caring in a corporate context. *Annual Review of Nursing Service, 11,* 4.

Marchette, L. & Halloman, F. (1986). Length of stay. *Journal of Nursing Administration, 16,* 12–19.

Maslow, A. (1968). *Toward a psychology of being.* New York: Harper & Row.

Mayer, D. (1987). Oncology nurses' versus cancer patients' perceptions of nurse caring behaviors: A replication study. *Oncology Nursing Forum, 14,* 48–52.

Mayerhoff, M. (1970). *On caring.* New York: Harper & Row.

Medicus Systems Corporation (1975). *The Medicus patient classification system.* Chicago: Author.

Merry, M. (1987). What is quality care? A model for measuring health care excellence. *Quarterly Review Bulletin, 10,* 2–4.

Miller-Bader, M. (1988). Nursing care behaviors that predict patient satisfaction. *Journal of Nursing Quality Assurance, 2,* 11–17.

Munson, F., Beckman, J., Clinton, J., Kever, C., & Simms, L. (1980). *Nursing assignment patterns: User's manual.* Washington, DC: AUPHA Press.

National Center for Health Statistics (1989). *Summary national hospital discharge survey advance data from vital and health statistics, 129,* No. (PHS) 88-1251, Hyattsville, MD: Public Health Service.

Nelson, C. & Goldstein, A. (1989). Health care quality: The new marketing challenge. *Health Care Management Review, 14,* 87–95.

Noddings, N. (1984). *Caring: A feminine approach to ethics and moral education.* Berkeley: University of California Press.

Norris, C. M. (1989). To care or not care—Questions! Questions! *Nursing and Health Care, 10,* 545–550.

Oberst, M. (1984). Patients' perceptions of care: Measurement of quality and satisfaction. *Cancer, 53,* 2366–2373.

Orlando, I. (1961). *The dynamic nurse patient relationship.* New York: George P. Putnam.

Orlick, S. (1988). The primacy of caring. *American Journal of Nursing, 259,* 318–319.

Pellegrino, E. (1985). Caring, curing, coping: Nurse, physician, patient relationships. In A. Bishop & J. R. Scudder (Eds.), *Health care ethics.* Birmingham, AL: University of Alabama Press, 8–30.

Proudfoot, M. (1983). Contagious calmness: A sense of calmness in acute care settings. *Topics in Clinical Nursing, 5,* 18–29.

Ray, M. (1987). Technological caring: A new model in critical care. *Dimensions of Critical Care Nursing, 6,* 166–173.

Reimen, D. J. (1986). Non-caring and caring in the clinical setting. *Topics in Clinical Nursing, 8,* 30–36.

Risser, N. (1975). Development of an instrument to measure patient satisfaction with nurses and nursing care in primary care settings. *Nursing Research, 24,* 45–52.

Roach, M. S. (1987). *The human act of caring: A blueprint for the health professionals.* Ontario, Canada: Canadian Hospital Association.

Rogers, C. (1969). The interpersonal relationship in the facilitation of learning. In S. Stoff & H. Schwartzberg (Eds.), *The human encounter.* New York: Harper & Row, 418–433.

Russakoff, S. (1987). Don't hospitals care anymore? *The Washington Post,* February 21.

Schaffer, P. L. (1987). Measuring nursing costs with patient acuity data. *Health Care Finance, 13,* 20–23.

Scott, W. R., Forrest, W. H., & Brown, B. (1976). Hospital structure and post-operative mortality and morbidity. In S. M. Shortell & M. Brown (Eds.), *Organizational research in hospitals.* Chicago: Blue Cross Association.

Spillane, R. (1987). Its great to have a caring nurse, if . . . *Nursing Management, 18,* 22.

Stevens, B. (1985). Tackling a changing society head on. *Nursing and Health Care, 6,* 27–30.

Travelbee, J. (1966). *Interpersonal aspects of nursing.* Philadelphia: F. A. Davis Company.

Walker, D. (1983). The cost of nursing care in hospitals. *Journal of Nursing Administration, 23,* 13–18.

Watson, J. (1979). *Nursing: The philosophy and science of caring.* Boulder: Colorado University Press.

Watson, J. (1985). *Nursing: Human science and human care.* Norwalk, CT: Appleton-Century-Crofts.

Watson, J. (1981). Some issues related to a science of caring for nursing practice. In M. M. Leininger (Ed.), *Caring: A human helping process.* Thorofare, NJ: Slack.

9

The Experience of Caring in the Acute Care Setting: Patient and Nurse Perspectives

Barbara Krainovich Miller
Judith Haber
Mary Woods Byrne

Theoreticians, researchers, educators, and practitioners across cultures recognize caring as an integral dimension of professional nursing (Benner, 1984; Gendron, 1988; Koldjeski, 1990; Leininger, 1984; Miller, Haber, & Byrne, 1990; Orem, 1985; Roach, 1984; Watson, 1988). Although theories on caring continue to be developed and research data become available, clarification of the concept remains a challenge.

Morse et al. (1990) recommend that essential to the refinement of caring theories is consideration of caring from the patient and nurse perspectives. Rawnsley (1990) proposes that caring as a construct requires clarification "if caring is to be considered a professional prerogative rather than a human attribute" (p. 41). According to Watson (1985a, 1988), one way to bring "caring" to the forefront of nursing practice and education is to clearly describe the phenomenon of caring in relation to nursing practice.

Contributors to *The Caring Imperative in Education* (Leininger & Watson, 1990), a collaborative publication of the University of Colorado Center for Human Caring and the International Association for Human Caring, support care as a concept central to nursing education and practice. Miller, Haber, and Byrne's (1990) study on caring in the student–teacher relationship suggests that teacher role modeling of caring behaviors not only maximizes the student's educational experience but also increases the likelihood that caring behaviors will be enacted in the practice setting.

There is a body of quantitative research related to the tasks of carrying out care as well. Such studies do not emanate from theoretical premises associated with caring theoreticians but focus instead on the tasks of providing care (Stevenson, 1990). The foci of several of these studies include: assessing and monitoring patient needs (Lindsey, 1983; Kim, 1987; Quall, 1988; Gordon, 1985), carrying out activities of care (Parsons & Kidd, 1989; Adams, 1986; Fenton, 1987), and non-invasive care modalities such as social support (Norbeck, 1988), biofeedback (Massey & Loomis, 1988), and guided imagery (Mast, 1986).

Qualitative research studies related to caring in the practice setting report a number of themes. Tripp-Reimer and Cohen's (1990) critical review of qualitative caring studies revealed these foci: the concept of care, the recipients of care, and lay and professional systems of care. These authors concluded that the majority of studies reviewed had design problems that reflected lack of methodological rigor in the qualitative tradition. Moreover, programs of caring research that would build the science of nursing in relation to caring were not evident except for the works of Aamodt (1978a,b, 1981, 1984, 1986), Leininger (1978a,b,c, 1981, 1984, 1985a, 1986), Morse (1983, 1987), and Morse and Park (1988). Despite the shortcomings that have been highlighted in the literature, the body of extant qualitative caring research must be recognized as having provided significant insights about the meaning of caring to the nursing profession (Tripp-Reimer & Cohen, 1990) as well as growing impetus for continuing research activity and refinement.

PURPOSE AND RESEARCH QUESTION

We conducted this phenomenological study to add to nursing's body of knowledge related to the experience of caring in the acute care setting from patient and nurse perspectives.

The following research question was asked: What is the lived experience of a caring nurse–patient interaction from the perspectives of nurses and hospitalized patients?

METHODOLOGY

Design Overview

As recommended by Streubert (1989, 1991), phenomenological analysis comprised the study methodology. According to Streubert (personal communication, September 26, 1991), she developed her method by an analysis and reformulation of the methods discussed by Colaizzi (1973, 1978), Giorgi (1985), Leininger (1985b), Oiler (1986), Paterson and Zderad (1976), Valle & King (1978), van Kaam (1966), and van Manen (1984). Specifically, we conducted phenomenological analysis of open-ended interviews with ongoing and post-data analysis of the interview data to: (1) identify themes of caring, (2) develop exhaustive descriptions of caring from the perspective of nurses and patients based on the identified themes, and (3) validate the exhaustive descriptions with the respective informants.

Data reliability was increased by our consistent format for conducting open-ended interviews. Saturation of themes cued researchers that sufficient data were collected. Three interviewers minimized the bias that each alone might bring to identification of themes. Informed consent was obtained. Confidentiality of the informants was assured.

Phenomenological research requires ongoing data analysis (Streubert, 1989). Miller, Haber, and Byrne's (1990) phenomenological study on caring in the educational setting used three researchers for collecting, processing, and synthesizing the data. Multiple researchers also act as consultants and provide a discussion forum for ongoing and post-data collection analysis. Miller, Haber, and Byrne recommended sessions between three to six hours for "dwelling together with the data" (p. 133). They highly and consistently recommended collaborative qualitative research endeavors.

Subjects and Setting

The study setting was a large metropolitan acute care medical center of a large eastern city of the United States. Approval was obtained for conducting the study from the institution's Human Subjects Review Board. A convenience sample of 15 patients and 16 nurses was drawn from three adult medical/surgical nursing care units. Patient selection criteria included patients who were oriented to time, place, and person, spoke English, and whose medical condition would not interfere with the interview. Selection criteria also included full-time registered nurses who spoke English and worked on the designated units. Nursing staff were asked to suggest patients who would be able to tolerate the interview process; conversely, the head nurse designated the registered nurses on the unit who were then asked to participate. Informed consent was obtained from the voluntary patient and nurse subjects. The interviews were conducted in a private area of the unit that was familiar to the informants.

Interview Format

Two open-ended questions were developed to begin the interview with each subject group. Patient informants were asked the following question: "Tell me about a caring nurse–patient interaction you have experienced." Nurse informants were asked: "Tell me about a patient interaction in which you provided caring." We developed guidelines for eliciting patient and nurse description of caring interactions so that each researcher would follow consistent guidelines for encouraging informants to explore thoughts on a caring interaction. For example, the interviewers might say, "go on, tell me more," "can you talk a little more about . . . ," or "can you give me an example."

We met prior to conducting the interviews and reviewed the interview guide protocol. Tape recorders with moveable microphones were secured and the equipment was pre-tested.

Procedure

The investigators and nursing administrators of the study institution determined that a clinical study of this nature would best be facilitated if each researcher was assigned to one of the study units. Informed consent was obtained. In addition, each informant's home address and telephone number was obtained in order that the study findings (exhaustive descriptions) could be sent to them for validation. Informants were asked to dwell on a caring patient–nurse interaction prior to the interview as well.

At the time of the taped open-end interview, the interviewer:

1. Reviewed the study's purpose.
2. Reviewed the consent form and elicited the informant's signature, home address, and telephone number.
3. Clarified any informant concerns.
4. Let informants practice using the equipment until they were ready to begin.
5. Initiated the interview by requesting that the patient-informant describe a situation in a patient–nurse interaction in which he or she experienced "caring" or requested that the nurse–informant describe a situation in which he or she gave care.
6. Encouraged informants to provide sufficient content for clarification.

With the completion of 12 patient interviews and 13 nurse interviews, saturation of data was reached. To ensure that we had not ended the interviews too soon, we conducted each one additional interview with another patient and nurse informant. Previously determined themes and patterns also emerged after these interviews were conducted.

ANALYSIS

Transcriptions of the audio-taped interviews were done initially To determine accuracy of the transcriptions, we read a transcription of the audio-taped interviews while listening to the tape. We reread the transcriptions a second time to gain further understanding of their meaning. We then identified caring statements and transcribed them onto index cards. After this process, we met to share and discuss identified caring statements. After several meetings, we merged caring statements and identified themes from the transcriptions. Once we identified themes, we wrote exhaustive descriptions of the phenomenon of caring experienced by the patient-informants and nurses during a patient–nurse interaction. Patient-informants and nurse informants were sent the respective descriptions for validation. They were asked if the written description captured the essence of their perception of a caring patient–nurse interaction. The informants were contacted by the principal investigator. They were requested to return an enclosed post card indicating their agreement or disagreement with the exhaustive description. We made follow-up phone calls as necessary. All nurse and patient informants who responded validated the exhaustive descriptions.

FINDINGS

Themes

The five parallel themes derived from the nurse and patient interviews follow: holistic understanding, connectedness/shared humanness, presence, anticipating and monitoring needs, and beyond the mechanical. These themes were used to write the exhaustive descriptions that the informants agreed captured the essence of a caring nurse-patient interaction.

Patient Exhaustive Description of a Caring Nurse-Patient Interaction

- Caring nurses are individuals who are concerned about you as a person and as a patient. Patients say caring nurses are interested in "all of you." They realize that the patient needs not only physical but emotional help; nurses take care of the whole environment, "including you."

- Caring nurses connect with you on a professional level but in a personal way. They greet you with a smile and look you in the eye when they talk. They ask you how you feel, how you slept, if the medication helped, is everything all right, and if you need anything. Because they really know you are a human being, apart from your tubes, your diabetes or your IV, they also ask about you, your family, your work, and your interests.

- Caring nurses are courteous, they call you by your name, they are kind, nice, never have a cross word and don't give you any aggravation. They come and see you, they stop for an extra minute, they spend time with you, they sit and listen. They take time with you when they do things. They display empathy by putting themselves in the patients' shoes. They remember what you've told them and make you feel like an important person.

- The caring nurse is always there to help and stays with you through the situation. They let you know it's okay to call, even for small things. When you ring they come quickly, even at night. They ask what you want and take care of what you want; that's very important, knowing they're always there to be of assistance. They do the best they can for you, if they can.

- Patients understand that caring nurses are human, too. Each has his or her own way of dealing with patients. They treat you as they would like to be treated. Patients know that even caring nurses have "off days"; but they still understand your moods. Just when you don't think they'll have time for you, they get there.

- Nurses take care of you in many ways. They anticipate your needs and meet them in advance. They're always watching; they make sure that everything's okay before there is a problem. They're right on top of things. They come in when the alarm goes off on the IV, not letting you sit there for a long time wondering. They make sure you don't have a high fever, they know when to wake you up to make sure you're okay, they organize your tests so you don't come back to a cold lunch. Caring nurses make sure you understand what is going to happen to you, they explain it over and over until you understand it.

- Caring nurses surround patients with consideration. They wake you gently in the morning, they are careful of the needles in your arm and are very nice and compassionate about giving physical care. Caring nurses know that when patients are very ill, they cannot help themselves and need to be helped as quickly as possible. They do the very basic things that are physically necessary like a bed bath or a bed pan. They offer to give you a backrub when you don't even think about needing one and then you're pleasantly surprised at how good it feels. They make you do the things that will help you get better even when you don't want to; like drinking a lot of water, getting out of bed and walking around or taking a medication in the middle of the night.

- Caring nurses know which of your needs to meet first. They know when the talking is most important, when your physical care is most important, and when you need to have both at the same time. Patients know which nurses understand how to do this because the care they give is not rote or mechanical.

Patients describe caring nurses as being ready to give of themselves; they seem to love being there and what they do satisfies them. Patients report they know that caring interactions make them feel better.

Nurse Exhaustive Description of a Caring
Nurse-Patient Interaction

From the nurse perspective, caring begins with holistic concern for the patient, including these aspects: the physical, the emotional, the spiritual, the family, and the environment. The caring never stops. Each day there is some amount of caring that nurses give their patients. Caring nurses recognize that not all patients are the same; they have individual needs. Therefore, it is essential for nurses to know their patients as people, to know them beyond their diagnosis and just what is written on the chart.

- Nurses describe caring as a way of being, an attitude, a personality that lets the patient know they care. Caring takes effort and energy; nurses have to feel good within themselves in order to transfer caring to their patients. Caring is loving, it's involved with everything. Nurses say each day you're giving love. Caring nurses respect the dignity of their patients. They give realistic encouragement and hope. They convey empathy as they strive to understand the patient's perspective. They treat their patients as they would like to be treated themselves. They share their patients' feelings, happy or sad; they can laugh or cry with them.

- Caring nurses establish relationships that are always professional but personal. They build rapport by introducing themselves, establishing eye contact, calling patients by their name, and, when they sense it's right, touching them. Caring nurses are available to their patients and concentrate on being there for them, even when rushed. They find the time to be there when patients need them most. They also know when patients need to talk or just have the nurse be there. They listen to them, they talk to them and they sit quietly with them. Even when patients can't talk, they talk to them and tune into their nonverbal responses. They tell patients when they will be there, when they will return, and who will be there in their place when they have a day off. They know that their presence is that important.

- Meeting the patients' physical needs provides an opportunity to get to know them. Giving a bed bath, a medication, or taking a blood pressure is done in a caring way when the nurse uses this time as an opportunity to talk and find out about the patient as a person. Nurses ask "what's happening today?" to check out the patient's understanding of their situation and correct any misunderstandings. Caring nurses explain procedures, medications, tests, and technical terms to patients and their families at their level as many times as needed so that they will understand what is happening to them. Nurses say that this builds trust between them and their patients.

- Caring nurses monitor their patients by simultaneously assessing, anticipating, prioritizing, and meeting their ever-changing needs. For nurses who really know their patients, sometimes they can tell "just by a look" what the patient's status is at that moment. Such nurses know, for example, when patients need to be given a bed bath or when they need to be pushed to do it for themselves. They know when to speak to the physician, the social worker, and nurse colleagues on the patients' behalf and when and how to enable patients to do this themselves. In this caring, nurses also include the family, preventing them from feeling like outsiders by helping them to understand and anticipate the course of the patient's progress—this makes all feel cared about.

- Caring practice has many outcomes for patients and nurses. Keeping patients involved in their care makes patients active participants who can initiate new tasks and routines and have a great impact on their rehabilitation. Caring results in patients' increased self-esteem and sense of trust. They feel good, relaxed, comfortable, happy, and important. In turn, nurses describe caring as providing them with a "magical" feeling of deep satisfaction that prompts them to love nursing. If you care, so nurses say, everything else falls right into place; indeed, both nurses and patients feel better.

Discussion of Exhaustive Descriptions

The exhaustive descriptions (findings) support a number of theories on caring as well as the findings of previous and recent qualitative studies. Patients and nurses value caring as an essential dimension of the recovery process. Similar to Watson (1985b), they value human care and like Leininger (1984) regard it as the essence of nursing. Informants consider caring as essential for human growth and survival (Leininger, 1981). Nurses express the idea that caring never stops; that every day there is some amount of caring they give their patients.

Orem (1985) differentiates between the specifics of taking care of and caring about. In the following passage, an informant implied validation of this perspective:

I was very cold and one of the nurses came in and said, "Gee, can I get you an extra blanket?" I said, "That would be terrific." And when she came back, she came not only with an extra blanket, she came back with a heated blanket! And she picked up all the blankets and put the warm blanket right next to me. And it was as if somebody had reached out and put me in her arms, so to speak, and it was a very, very, comforting thing.

Benner's (1984) study, differentiating novice from expert practitioners, revealed the following six different qualities of power associated with caring: transformative power, integrative caring, advocacy, healing power, participative/affirmative power, and problem solving. The findings, as indicated in the exhaustive descriptions, closely support Benner's theory. While this study was not observational, relying instead on self-report data to capture the lived experience of caring, all nurses did perceive caring to be a philosophical perspective embedded in their practice. Certainly, we do not know if these nurses practice according to their stated philosophy; future studies are needed to clarify this issue (Tripp-Reimer & Cohen, 1990). Although not all of the nurse informants would meet Benner's chronological criteria of an expert nurse, all nurses did express the centrality of intuition and anticipation in "just knowing when a patient needs what, when and from whom." To these nurses, this was caring.

The findings specifically support Riemen's (1986) pioneering study on the essential structure of caring interactions between nurses and patients. Other caring studies by Drew (1986), Paternoster (1988), and Larson (1987), Swanson (1990), and Sherwood (1988) support the finding of Riemen's study as well as the present study. All of these studies suggest that caring is one of the key components of patient well being. The parallel themes of this study, holistic understanding, connectedness/shared humanness, presence, anticipation and monitoring of patient needs, and beyond the mechanical, are all reflected in the previous studies.

IMPLICATIONS AND RECOMMENDATIONS

Research

Concept clarification directed at uncovering and describing the common essences of caring in the practice setting will facilitate further development of a scientific body of knowledge related to caring (Norbeck & Woods, 1990; Watson, 1990). However, clinical studies need to focus on patients in order to place "Caring in a meaning-intensive clinical context . . ." (Swanson, 1990, p. 70). Furthermore, replication of nurse–patient caring studies, using patients at different lifecycle stages, experiencing acute, critical and chronic illnesses, will clarify the concept of caring as lived by patients.

Both qualitative and quantitative clinical studies also are needed to promote concept clarification. To this date, in the research conducted from both paradigms Stevenson (1990) and Tripp-Reimer and Cohen (1990) note a certain lack of methodological rigor. These researchers suggest that descriptive quantitative studies include patients as expert panelists when establishing instrument content validity. We must remember that validating study findings with informants is an essential step in phenomenological methodology

(Swanson, 1990), as well as other types of qualitative research. Such validation should not be overlooked.

Nurse Self-Care

Baillie, Trygstad, and Cordoni (1989) and Benner (1984), in their studies on nurse burnout, suggest that self-care influences the nurse's ability to care for and about others. Unfortunately, there is a paucity of data related to the importance of self-care (Benner, 1984; Leininger, 1988) in the caring literature.

Although findings of the current study in regard to nurse self-care may sound simplistic, in fact, they provide an elegant and powerful context in which to consider nurse self-care. The process of caring in the acute care setting would be strengthened by focusing first on nurses' self-care. It is important for nurses to start caring for themselves. Although caring for self is, of course, an individual process, it always involves taking sufficient time to focus on self. Several examples of "taking time for oneself" are: leaving the unit for a mid-morning "break," a meal, scheduling a vacation, learning relaxation techniques, doing aerobics, setting limits on the number of tasks one agrees to, or even taking the time to window shop or go to a movie. In other words, we are advocating taking the time to make and keep appointments with one's self.

Another aspect of "nurse self-care" is engaging in self-praise. Benner (1984) contends that nurses always have a story to tell. Nurses' stories involve nurses telling other nurses about their patients and all the interventions performed. But, most importantly, the talk is about the caring acts they performed in relation to nursing intervention, and how wonderful this made them and their patients feel. Benner's (1989a,b,c,d, 1990) series of commentaries on nurses's stories (e.g., Ball, 1989; Dyck, 1989; Gruber, 1989; McNall, 1989; Stewart, 1989; Stephany, 1990), which appeared in the *American Journal of Nursing,* are excellent examples of nurses sharing their unique caring stories in formal written communication with those in the health care discipline. Kraegel and Kachoyeanos' (1989) *Just a Nurse* is another wonderful example of nurses sharing their paradigm cases with not only other nurses but with the lay community who are all too often unaware of the real work of nurses.

Nurses' story-telling is not only a healing process for nurses and patients, but enjoins powerful expressive process in and of itself. One of Benner's (1984) qualities of power associated with the caring provided by nurses is referred to as "participative/affirmative power." Although Benner would agree that some of the previously described "taking time for oneself" activities are important, she does not believe that nurses will protect themselves against burnout by simply distancing themselves from caring situations. Nurses' story-telling can help nurses reframe their work activities by using "the meaning and resources inherent in . . . [these] poignant event[s]" (p. 214) to reactivate the sorely needed "precious juices of caring" (p. 213). We further suggest that nurses who are able to care for themselves are better able to offer the type of caring described so beautifully by the nurses and patients of this study and which, as implied by patient informants, leads to patient satisfaction.

Total Institutional Commitment

We suggest that an institution's philosophy include a commitment to promoting the role of care. The following are but a few examples of how, at the nursing departmental level, care behaviors could be infused:

1. Interviews with potential nurse employees would include matching their philosophy of caring with the institution's, as well as eliciting their examples of specific care behaviors.
2. Orientation and staff development programs would overtly address the institution's philosophy of caring; caring behaviors would be taught with the same emphasis as a technical skill.

3. Developing objective quantitative criteria for raises and promotion based on the institution's philosophy of care.

A department of nursing's research or quality management committee could assist in bringing to fruition these recommendations. An ad hoc committee could be formed which would consist of staff and administrative level nurses and patients. This committee could:

1. Survey nurses and patients for the purpose of identifying "caring" nurses.
2. Conduct interviews with the designated caring nurses for their views on what constitutes caring behaviors.
3. Perform direct observations of designated caring nurses during interactions with patients.

The retrieved data could assist in validating and refining the department of nursing's caring philosophy and related caring behaviors. In turn, care evaluation and patient satisfaction tools could be developed and then validated using a panel of experts comprised of patients and nurses.

CONCLUSION

In general, the findings and implementation of the recommendations from this study will add to nursing's growing body of knowledge on caring, as well as help to legitimize and assist others in "valuing the caring practices and expert knowledge embedded in nursing practice" (Benner & Wrubel, 1989, p. xv–xvi). It also will lend support to leaders in care giving professions who are trying to develop "models of professionalism that improve care givers' status, without compromising the heart of their work—care. . . . [and] develop new, relationship-oriented, caring models of professionalism that also 'keep the marketplace in its place'" (Gordon, 1991, p. 48).

REFERENCES

Aamodt, A. (1978a). Socio-cultural dimensions of caring in the world of the Papago child and adolescent. In M. M. Leininger (Ed.), *Transcultural nursing: Concepts, theories, and practices.* New York: John Wiley & Sons, 239–250.

Aamodt, A. (1978b). The care component in a health and healing system. In E. Bauwens (Ed.), *The anthropology of health.* St. Louis: C.V. Mosby.

Aamodt, A. (1981). Neighboring: Discovering support systems among Norwegian-American women. In D. Messerschmidt (Ed.), *Anthropologists at home: Toward an anthropology of issues in America.* New York: Cambridge University Press, 133–149.

Aamodt, A. (1984). Themes and issues in conceptualizing care. In M. M. Leininger (Ed.), *Care: The essence of nursing and health.* Thorofare, NJ: Slack, 75–79.

Aamodt, A. (1986). Discovering the child's view of alopecia: Doing ethnography. In P. L. Munhall & C. J. Oiler (Eds.), *Nursing research: A qualitative perspective.* Norwalk, CT: Appleton-Century-Crofts, 163–172.

Adams, M. (1986). Aging: Gerontological nursing research. In J. J. Fitzpatrick, R. L. Taunton & J. Q. Beneliel (Eds.), *Annual review of nursing research: Volume 4.* New York: Springer, 77–103.

Baillie, V. K., Trygstad, L., & Cordoni, T. I. (1989). *Effective nursing leadership: A practical guide.* Rockville, Maryland.

Ball, B. (1989). Simplifying care. *American Journal of Nursing, 89*(11), 1466–1467.

Benner, P. (1984). *From novice to expert: Excellence and power in clinical nursing.* Menlo Park, CA: Addison-Wesley.

Benner, P. (1989a). Commentary. *American Journal of Nursing, 89*(4), 503.

Benner, P. (1989b). Commentary. *American Journal of Nursing, 89*(6), 825.

Benner, P. (1989c). Commentary. *American Journal of Nursing, 89*(9), 1163.

Benner, P. (1989d). Commentary. *American Journal of Nursing, 89*(11), 1468.

Benner, P. (1990). Commentary. *American Journal of Nursing, 90*(4), 56.

Benner, P., & Wrubel, J. (1989). *The primacy of caring: Stress and coping in health and illness.* Reading, MA: Addison-Wesley.

Colaizzi, P. F. (1978). Psychological research as the phenomenologist views it. In R. Valle & M. King (Eds.), *Existential-phenomenological alternatives for psychology.* New York: Oxford University Press.

Colaizzi, P. F. (1973). *Reflections and research in psychology: A phenomenological study of learning.* Dubuque, IA: Kendall-Hunt.

Drew, N. (1986). Exclusion and confirmation: A phenomenology of patient's experiences with caregivers. *Image 18*, 39–43.

Dyck, B. (1989). Dialogue with excellence: The paper crane. *American Journal of Nursing, 89*(6), 824–825.

Fenton, M. V. (1987). Development of the scale of humanistic nursing behaviors. *Nursing Research, 36*, 82–87.

Gendron, D. (1988). The expressive form of caring. *Perspectives in caring monograph 2.* Faculty of Nursing, University of Toronto.

Giorgi, (1985). *Phenomenology and psychological research.* Pittsburgh, PA: Duquesne University Press.

Gordon, M. (1985). Nursing diagnosis. In H. H. Werley & J. J. Fitzpatrick (Eds.), *Annual review of nursing research: Volume 3.* New York: Springer, 127–146.

Gordon, S. (1991). Fear of caring: The feminist paradox. *American Journal of Nursing, 91*(2), 44–48.

Gruber, M. (1989). A dialogue with excellence: The power of certainty. *American Journal of Nursing, 89*(4), 502–503.

Kim, M. J. (1987). Physiological responses in health and illness: an overview. In J. J. Fitzpatrick & R. L. Taunton (Eds.), *Annual review of nursing research: Volume 5.* New York: Springer, 79–104.

Koldjeski, D. (1990). Toward a theory of professional nursing caring: A unifying perspective. In M. M. Leininger & J. Watson (Eds.), *The caring imperative in education.* New York: National League for Nursing, 45–57.

Kraegel, R. N., & Kachoyeanos, R. N. (1989). *Just a nurse.* New York: Dutton.

Larson, P. (1987). Comparison of cancer patients' and professional nurses' perceptions of important nurse caring behaviors. *Heart and Lung, 16*, 187–193.

Leininger, M. M. (1978a). Transcultural nursing: A new and scientific subfield of study in nursing. In M. M. Leininger (Ed.), *Transcultural nursing: Concepts, theories, and practices.* New York: John Wiley & Sons.

Leininger, M. M. (1978b). Transcultural nursing theories and research approaches. In M. M. Leininger (Ed.), *Transcultural nursing: Concepts, theories, and practices.* New York: John Wiley & Sons.

Leininger, M. M. (1978c). Toward conceptualization of transcultural health care systems: Concepts and a model. In M. M. Leininger, (Ed.), *Transcultural nursing: Concepts, theories, and practices.* New York: John Wiley & Sons, 53–74.

Leininger, M. M. (1981). Cross-cultural hypothetical functions of caring and nursing care. In M. M. Leininger, (Ed.), *Caring: An essential human need.* Thorofare, NJ: Slack.

Leininger, M. M. (1984). Care: The essence of nursing and health. In M. M. Leininger, (Ed.), *Caring: The essence of nursing and health*, Thorofare, NJ: Slack.

Leininger, M. M. (1985a). Ethnography and ethnonursing: Models and modes of qualitative data analysis. In M. M. Leininger (Ed.), *Qualitative research methods in nursing*. Orlando, FL: Grune & Stratton, 33–71.

Leininger, M. M. (1985b). *Qualitative research methods in nursing*. Orlando, FL: Grune & Stratton.

Leininger, M. M. (1986). Care facilitation and resistance factors in the culture of nursing. *Topics in Clinical Nursing, 8,* 1–12.

Leininger, M. M. (Ed.). (1988). *Care: Discovery and uses in clinical and community nursing*. Detroit: Wayne State University Press.

Leininger, M. M., & Watson, J. (Eds.). (1990). *The caring imperative in education*. New York: National League for Nursing.

Lindsey, A. M. (1983). Phenomena and physiological variables of relevance to nursing: Review of a decade of work, part II. *Western Journal of Nursing Research, 5,* 40–63.

Massey, J., & Loomis, M. (1988). When should nurses use research findings? *Applied Nursing Research, 1*(1), 32–40.

Mast, D. E. (1986). Effects of imagery. *Image, 18,* 118–120.

McNall, C. C. (1989). Healing we cannot explain. *American Journal of Nursing, 89*(9), 1162–1163.

Miller, B. K., Haber, J., & Byrne, M. W. (1990). The experience of caring in the teaching-learning process of nursing education: Student and teacher. In M. M. Leininger & J. Watson (Eds.). *The caring imperative in education*. New York: National League for Nursing, 125–135.

Morse, J. (1983). An ethnoscientific analysis of comfort: A preliminary investigation. *Nursing Papers/Perspectives in Nursing, 15,* 6–19.

Morse, J. (1987). The meaning of health in an inner city community (research). *Nursing Papers, 19*(2), 27–40.

Morse, J., Park, C. (1988). Home birth and hospital deliveries: A comparison of the perceived painfulness of parturition. *Research in Nursing and Health, 11*(3), 175–81.

Morse, J., Solberg, S. M., Neander, W. L., Bottorff, J. L., & Johnson, J. L. (1990). Concepts of caring and caring as a concept. *Advances in Nursing Science, 13*(1), 1–14.

Norbeck, J. (1988). Social support. In J. J. Fitzpatrick, R. L. Taunton, & J. Q. Beneliel (Eds.), *Annual review of nursing research: Volume 6* (pp. 85–128). New York: Springer.

Norbeck, J., & Woods, N. F. (1990). Summary and synthesis of small group deliberations. In J. S. Stevenson & T. Tripp-Reimer (Eds.), *Knowledge about care and caring: State of the art and future developments.* St. Louis, MO: American Academy of Nursing, 145–146.

Oiler, C. J. (1986). Qualitative methods: Phenomenology. In P. Moccia (Ed.), *New approaches to theory development.* New York: National League for Nursing, 74–103.

Orem, D. (1985). *Nursing: Concepts of practice.* (3rd ed.). Chevy Chase, MD: McGraw-Hill.

Parsons, L. C. & Kidd, P. S. (1989). Neurologic nursing research. In J. J. Fitzpatrick, R. L. Taunton & J. Q. Beneliel (Eds.), *Annual review of nursing research: Volume 7.* New York: Springer, 3–25.

Paternoster, J. (1988). How patients know that nurses care about them. *The Journal, 19*(4), 17–21.

Paterson, J. G., & Zderad, L. T. (1976). *Humanistic nursing.* New York: John Wiley & Sons.

Quall, S. J. (1988). Hemodynamic monitoring: A review of the literature. *Applied Nursing Research, 1,* 58–67.

Rawnsley, M. (1990). Of human bonding: The context of nursing as caring. *Advances in Nursing Science, 13*(1), 41–48.

Riemen, D. (1986). The essential structure of a caring interaction: Doing phenomenology. In P. Munhall & C. J. Oiler, *Nursing research: A qualitative perspective.* Norwalk, CT: Appleton-Century-Crofts, 85–108.

Roach, M. (Ed.). (1984). *Caring: The human mode of being.* Toronto: University of Toronto.

Sherwood, G. D. (1988). *Nurses' caring as perceived by post-operative patients: A phenomenology study.* Unpublished doctoral dissertation, University of Texas at Austin.

Stephany, T. M. (1990). Dialogue with excellence: A death in the family. *American Journal of Nursing, 90*(4), 54–56.

Stevenson, J. S. (1990). Quantitative care research: Review of content, process and product. In J. S. Stevenson & T. Tripp-Reimer. *Knowledge about care and caring: State of the art and future developments.* St. Louis, MO: American Academy of Nursing, 97–118.

Stewart, P. B. (1989). A moment of truth. *American Journal of Nursing, 89*(11), 1467–1468.

Streubert, H. J. (1989). *A description of clinical experience as perceived by clinical nurse educators and students.* Unpublished doctoral dissertation, Teachers College, Columbia University.

Streubert, H. J. (1991). Phenomenologic research as a theoretic initiative in community health nursing. *Public Health Nursing, 8,* 119–123.

Swanson, K. M. (1990). Providing care in the NICU: Sometimes an act of love. *Advances in Nursing Science, 13*(1), 60–73.

Tripp-Reimer, T., & Cohen, M. Z. (1990). Qualitative approaches to care: A critical review. In J. S. Stevenson & T. Tripp-Reimer (Eds.), *Knowledge about care and caring: State of the art and future developments.* St. Louis, MO: American Academy of Nursing, 83–96.

Valle, R. S., & King, M. (1978). *Existential phenomenological alternatives for psychology.* New York: Oxford Press.

van Kaam, A. (1966). *Existential foundations of psychology.* New York: University Press of America.

van Manen, M. (1984). Practicing phenomenological writing. *Phenomenology and Pedagogy, 2*(1), 36–72.

Watson, J. (1985a). Nursing: A human science and human care. In J. Watson (Ed.), *A theory of nursing.* Norwalk, CT: Appleton-Century-Crofts.

Watson, J. (1985b). Reflecting on different methodologies for the future of nursing. In M. M. Leininger (Ed.), *Qualitative research in methods in nursing.* Orlando, FL: Grune & Stratton, 343–349.

Watson, J. (1988). Human caring as moral context for nursing education. *Nursing & Health Care, 9*(8), 422–425.

Watson, J. (1990). Caring knowledge and informed moral passion. *Advances in Nursing Science, 13*(1), 15–24.

10

Trust as a Caring Construct with the Critically Ill: A Beginning Exploration

Catherine Snelson

Trust as a care construct is embedded in the nurse-client relationship in critical care. In this paper, I will analyze the current literature and propose a method for explication of the meanings of the domain of trust in the critical care nurse-client relationship from an emic perspective. In the context of such a short and intense relationship frequently experienced in critical care, it is imperative that critical care nurses quickly understand the patient's perspective of trust in order to implement professional nursing care.

Development of a professional nurse-client relationship is an essential component toward full attainment of the goals of professional nursing. Without the establishment of this relationship, interactions between the nurse and the client are a facade rather than a productive encounter where both parties establish a framework from which to grow. According to Bevis (1988), caring helps to ". . . raise human relationships to satisfying experiences of pleasure, security, trust, growth, and positive activity" (p. 49).

As a construct, trust is often used in the nursing literature when discussing the formation of a therapeutic nurse-client relationship. As Moore and Hartman (1988) have stated: "Therapeutic relationships imply the establishment of a warm, trusting relationship between the nurse and client for the purpose of helping the client" (p. 92). Trust can bridge the gap between the nurse and the client in the relationship (Thomas, 1978). In a very thoughtful and imaginative monograph, Gendron (1988) describes the phases of the nurse-patient relationship. The introductory phase describes trust as an important task. Trust ". . . makes the regularity of reliability and consistency a strong theme" (p. 26). Trust then provides for the positive underpinnings of the caregiver to enhance this phase of the nurse-patient relationship.

Trust, by the critically ill patient of the nurse, is important for assisting the patient to regain and maintain an optimal level of health in the context of a critical life-threatening illness. When trust is present, the patient can channel valuable emotional energy into achieving the goal of optimal health, instead of wondering about and doubting the quality of nursing care and information communicated. Beard (1982) examined the relationship between interpersonal trust, life events, and coronary heart disease risk factors. Beard conceptualized trust as an internal factor that helps to defend the body against stresses. Beard hypothesized that in situations when there are alterations in the levels of trust, the general adaptation syndrome is activated. If unresolved, there is depletion of resources necessary for homeostasis. Beard's study revealed a statistically significant correlation between interpersonal trust and life events. These findings suggest that interpersonal trust is an important variable influencing neurophysiological adaptation to stress from life events. If the level of interpersonal trust can be increased, then the adaptation syndrome response to stress can be decreased.

Trust that is explicit in nature implies it is not automatic, but rather, according to Gadow (1985), occurs when the patient is willing to offer the professional in the relationship a gift, ". . . a gift of inestimable value, without which even the most one-sided relationship collapses; the gift of trust" (p. 42). Viewed in this sense, trust is defined by the client and his or her worldview, lifeways, values, and beliefs and is therefore unique to that client and that particular nurse-client relationship.

Several key questions should be considered by nurses when exploring the meanings of trust from the emic perspective: Is trust explicit in the nurse-client relationship? Does the patient implicitly trust the nurse because the nurse is a member of the nursing profession? Can the client in principle trust nurses he or she has never met to provide care in a critical care situation? Can the nurse assume that in this relationship the client trusts without question?

OVERVIEW OF THE DOMAIN

To better understand the concept of trust and its theoretical applications, I reviewed scholarly literature related to trust for the discovery of its ontologic and epistemologic development.

Erikson (1963) defines basic trust as a general state of reliance on others and self. Erikson identifies the need for maternal caring to develop this sense of basic trust in self and the world. The amount of trust derived from such infant experiences depends on the quality of the maternal relationship.

Bevis (1988) identifies the need for the development of both autonomy and trust as the basis for a true caring relationship. If either autonomy or trust is skipped, truly caring relationships cannot develop.

Rotter (1967) defines interpersonal trust ". . . as an expectancy held by an individual that the word, promise, verbal, or written statement of another individual or group can be relied on [*sic*]" (p. 65). Wheeless and Grotz (1977) summarized interpersonal trust as a process of holding favorable perceptions of another, which produce certain dependent behaviors in a risky situation, where the outcomes dependent upon the other person are not known.

Trust also can be conceptualized as a specific trust or trust in a specific individual rather than others in general. Wheeless and Grotz (1977) defined individualized trust as trust in a specific person or the perceived trustworthiness of a target person.

As a result of extensive Culture Care theory research of 54 cultures, Leininger (1991) has derived 172 care/caring constructs. These constructs are derived wholly from an emic perspective and typify behavioral attributes representative of caring. Leininger has identified trust as one of these care constructs.

Watson (1985) states that "of all the problems that can arise in nursing care, perhaps the most common is failure to establish rapport or a helping-trust relationship with the other person" (p. 25). Watson believes that a patient who feels the nurse really cares about the person and understands the person's individual needs and concerns is likely to establish trust, faith, and hope in the nursing care. Furthermore, Watson believes a helping-trust relationship is a basic element for high quality care. Some of the attitudinal processes nurses must bring to this relationship, which have been empirically validated, are: congruence or genuineness; empathy, or the ability of the nurse to experience the other's private world; and non-possessive warmth. Boyle (1988) believes that trust in itself is not a single function, but with certain qualities exhibited by the nurse such as genuineness, empathy, and acceptance, facilitates a trusting client relationship.

Cronin and Harrison (1988) measured patient perceptions of nurse caring behaviors for post-myocardial infarction with the Caring Behaviors Assessment (CBA). The CBA was ordered in seven subscales congruent with Watson's (1985) carative factors. The nursing behaviors perceived as most indicative of caring by patients focused on the Human Needs Assistance subscale or the monitoring of patient condition and the demonstration of professional competence. The Helping/Trust subscale was ranked sixth in importance by patients as an important caring behavior after myocardial infarction. The development of a caring relationship and the experience of trust as the basis of the relationship can be enhanced if expert nursing care is provided and patients' basic physical needs are met. Brown (1986) states that patient confidence in the nurses' ability to meet physical care needs is fundamental to the experience of care. As professional competency is demonstrated, more expressive activities, such as trust become more important.

Roach (1984) has identified the "Five C's" as attributes of professional caring: compassion, competence, confidence, conscience and commitment. As defined by Roach, the attribute of confidence is that quality that fosters trusting relationships. "Caring confidences foster trust without dependency; communicates truth without violence; and creates a relationship of respect without paternalism, or without engendering a response born out of fear or powerlessness. Confidence, then, is a critical attribute of professional caring" (p. 24).

Boyle (1988) defines trust ". . . as that relationship wherein the patient or client has confidence or faith in the nurse" (p. 44). As a result of this confidence the patient ". . . relies upon the nurses' integrity to accept him, his feelings, and needs and to provide nursing care based on knowledge skill and expertise" (p. 44). It is Boyle's belief that clients must have trust and confidence in the person helping them in order to be "cared for."

Bergbom-Engberg and Haljamae (1988) conducted a retrospective study on the influence of nursing care related factors on the experience of security or insecurity by critically ill patients during ventilator treatment. A particularly important reason for feeling secure was due to the presence of a nurse who could be trusted (34%). Lack of trust in the nurse on duty (24%) and an inability to trust the technical equipment (36%) were cited as primary reasons for patient insecurity.

Larson (1987) conducted an investigation of both patient and nurse perceptions of nurse caring behaviors, with the Caring Assessment Instrument (CARE-Q) used to determine perceptions. The CARE-Q consists of 50 nurse caring behaviors ordered in six subscales with trusting relationships identified as one of the six subscales. Nurses perceived comforting and trusting relationship behaviors as being most important in making patients feel cared for. In contrast, cancer patients perceived accessibility, monitoring, and following through as the most important caring behaviors. The only item that both patients and nurses agreed with as an important caring behavior came from the Trusting Relationship subscale. The specific item for this subscale identified as important by both patients and nurses was "Puts patient first, no matter what" (p. 191).

Utilizing the method of structural conceptualization, Valentine (1989) asked nurses, patients, and nurse theorists/researchers to conceptualize caring in a nursing context. A separate concept map was derived for each group. Items common to all three groups were warmth, acceptance, kindness, trust, and compassion. As identified by the patients, nurse qualities that increased trust were friendliness, competence, and confidence.

Ray (1987), utilizing the phenomenologic research procedure to study human caring in critical care, posed one central question to eight critical care nurses: "What is the meaning of caring to you in the critical care unit?" (p. 167). Five themes were identified from their responses. One of the themes included the statement: "Caring is trust among patients, families, nurses, and physicians" (p. 168).

The scholarly literature has offered many dimensions within which to conceptualize the meaning of trust. Specifically, nursing literature is replete with etic meanings of trust and professional nursing care that facilitates the development of trust in the nurse-client relationship. Unfortunately, very little literature was found that explicated emic meanings of trust in this relationship or specific patterns of care that enhanced the development of patient trust. The ontology of trust is overwhelmingly derived from the etic perspective.

THEORETICAL FRAMEWORK

Leininger's theory of Cultural Care Diversity and Universality (1988b) offers the theoretical framework for exploration of the emic meaning of the care construct *trust* in the nurse-client relationship in critical care. Leininger states that cultural care provides a means to study and predict nursing knowledge and care practice. The goal of the theory is to generate new knowledge and identify ways to provide culture congruent nursing care practices. All acutely ill patients in a hospitalized setting will be viewed as the major culture. Within this culture there are subgroups or smaller group (Leininger, 1990). The subculture is defined as those adult patients who are critically ill and hospitalized in a critical care unit.

The Sunrise model is used to depict the theory. Three dominant modes in the Sunrise model that guide nursing decisions to provide culturally congruent care are culture care preservation/maintenance; culture care accommodation/negotiation; and culture care repatterning/restructuring. Trust as embedded in the process of an actual caring occasionally is predicted to effect all three modes. However, there also are factors identified as part of the social structure and worldview of the Sunrise model that influence care and health patterns and expressions of human beings. While still focusing on the interaction between the professional and folk systems, these factors also may influence the development of trust and need to be considered. Examples of these factors include: technological, religious and philosophical, kinship and social, cultural values and beliefs, political and legal, and economic and educational factors.

RESEARCH METHODOLOGY

In studying trust, the researcher should use the qualitative research methodology of ethnonursing. This qualitative methodology allows the researcher to obtain and reveal the emic perspective of trust in the critical care unit. Much current research on trust has utilized only quantitative scales. However, quantitatively derived variables/statements may not accurately reflect the client's perspective of trust or those patterns of care that influence the development of trust in the nurse-client relationship in critical care. It is the researcher's goal to address the following research questions:

- What are the emic meanings of trust as it relates to a caring relationship in critical care?
- What are the characteristics of trust in this relationship?
- Does trust enhance the nature of a caring relationship as perceived by the patient in critical care?
- What patterns of care, defined by the patient, foster the development of trust by the patient of the nurse in critical care?

DISCUSSION

Trust is an essential component of a professional nurse-client relationship in critical care. The presence of trust in this relationship, at the very least, provides the client with assurance of safe, competent nursing care. This assurance is an essential ingredient for enhancing client recovery. The client's basic trust of self and the world has not only been undermined, the essence of the client's being has been most intimately threatened with a life-threatening illness or injury. A critical care nurse perceived by the client to be trustworthy may be all the critically ill client sees as the difference between life and death. In this sense, trust is defined by the client and is unique to that particular nurse-client relationship.

Leininger (1988a) hypothesizes there must be congruence between the care giver and care recipient's behaviors and goals. This congruence is important for therapeutic practices to occur. Furthermore, if the nurse as the professional care giver lacks knowledge about the cultural beliefs, values, and practices of caring, this can produce stresses and conflicts for the client. As a manifestation of expressive caring, trust will not be therapeutic for the patient if there is not congruence in meaning between the nurse and client. Questions a researcher might consider asking the patient to derive the emic meanings of trust and answer the research questions posed by this proposal include:

1. Tell me about your relationship with the nurses who have taken care of you in critical care?
2. What nursing activities did a specific nurse do that helped you feel confident in your relationship with that nurse?
3. What did the nurse do to help you feel you could rely on the nurse when you were a patient in critical care?
4. What nursing activities helped you to feel safe during the time you were in critical care?

A specific inquiry guide, focused on trust phenomena, also might be developed for use by the researcher as an enabler during this study.

The greater the efforts of the professional nurse to blend folk caring practices with professional care practices, the greater the client's satisfaction (Leininger, 1988a). Therefore, it is the responsibility of the critical care nurse to have a most intimate understanding of the emic meanings of the care construct trust. The critical care nurse must then apply that understanding to the development

of a trusting nurse-client relationship and delivery of culturally congruent professional nursing care.

REFERENCES

Andersson-Segesten, K. (1991). Patient's experience of uncertainty in illness in two intensive coronary units. *Scandinavian Journal of Caring
Science, 5*(1), 43–47.

Beard, M. (1982). Trust, life events, and risk factors among adults. *Advances
in Nursing Science, 4*(4), 26–43.

Bergbom-Engberg, I., & Haljamae, H. (1988). A retrospective study of
patient's recall of respirator treatment (2): Nursing care factors and
feelings of security/insecurity. *Intensive Care Nursing, 4*, 95–101.

Bevis, E. O. (1988). Caring: A life force. In M. M. Leininger (Ed.), *Caring, an
essential human need*. Detroit: Wayne State University Press, 49–59.

Boyle, J. (1988). An application of the structural-functional method to the
phenomenon of caring. In M. M. Leininger (Ed.), *Caring, an essential
human need*. Detroit: Wayne State University Press, 37–47.

Brown, L. (1986). The experience of care, patient perspectives. *TCN, 8*(2),
56–63.

Cronin, S. N., & Harrison, B. (1988). Importance of nurse caring behaviors
as perceived by patients after myocardial infarction. *Heart & Lung,
17*(4), 374–380.

Erikson, E. (1963). *Childhood and society* (2nd ed.). New York: W. W. Norton.

Gadow, S. A. (1985). Nurse and patient: The caring relationship. In A. H.
Bishop & J. R. Scudder, Jr. (Eds.), *Caring curing coping nurse physician
patient relationships*. University, AL: The University of Alabama Press,
31–43.

Gendron, D. (1988). *The expressive form of caring* (Perspective in Caring
Monograph 2). Toronto: University of Toronto, Faculty of Nursing.

Larson, P. J. (1987). Comparison of cancer patients' and professional nurses'
perception of important nurse caring behaviors. *Heart & Lung, 16*(2),
187–192.

Leininger, M. M. (1988a). The phenomenon of caring: Importance,
research questions and theoretical considerations. In M. M. Leininger
(Ed.), *Caring, an essential human need*. Detroit: Wayne State University Press, 3–16.

Leininger, M. M. (1988b). Leininger's theory of nursing: Cultural care diversity and universality. *Nursing Science Quarterly 1* (4), 152–160.

Leininger, M. M. (1990). The significance of cultural concepts in nursing. *Journal of Transcultural Nursing, 2*(1), 52–59.

Leininger, M. M. (1991). N820 Human Care Seminar Handout. Wayne State University. Summer 1991.

Moore, J. C., & Hartman, C. R. (1988). Developing a therapeutic relationship. In C. K. Beck, R. P. Rawlins, & S. R. Williams (Eds.), *Mental health-psychiatric nursing* (2nd ed.). St. Louis: C. V. Mosby, 92–117.

Ray, M. A. (1987). Technological caring: A new model in critical care. *Dimensions of Critical Care Nursing, 6*(3), 166–173.

Roach, M. S. (1984). *Caring: The human mode of being implications for nursing* (Perspective of Caring Monograph 1). Toronto: University of Toronto, Faculty of Nursing.

Rotter, J. B. (1967). A new scale for the measurement of interpersonal trust. *Journal of Personality, 35*(4), 651–665.

Thomas, M. D. (1978). Trust. In C. E. Carlson & B. Blackwell (Eds.), *Behavioral concepts and nursing interventions* (2nd ed.). Philadelphia: J. B. Lippincott, 164–170.

Valentine, K. (1989). Contributions to the theory of care. *Evaluation and Program Planning, 12,* 17–23.

Watson, J. (1985). *The philosophy and science of caring.* Boulder, CO: Colorado Associated University Press.

Wheeless, L. R., & Grotz, J. (1977). The measurement of trust and its relationship to self disclosure. *Human Communication Research, 3*(3), 250–257.

11

Mothers and Drugs: Two Possibilities for Caring

Toni M. Vezeau

In this paper, I deal with a clinical situation seen commonly today: that of the breastfeeding mother who ingests drugs. The complexity of this situation involves both legal and health issues, and bears directly upon the relationship between a mother and her child.

Health care providers believe that their caring can offer direction to clinical decision making. However, *caring* can have variant meanings (Vezeau & Schroeder, 1991). If caring is to offer a rudder in ethical dilemmas, clinicians must be certain of the assumptions and implications of the caring philosophy being adopted.

Here, I will explore two models of caring, as developed by Nel Noddings (1984) and Susan Griffin (1978) in a narrative written about John James Audubon, in light of mothers and drugs. Each caring approach will show differences in the methods of knowing, in the choice of options, and in the forms for action for all participants.

CONFLICT: MOTHERS AND DRUGS

The following passage is from a true story, in which names have been changed but not the dilemma.

> *Latoya was thrilled about her newborn baby girl, Crystal. Although her pregnancy had not been planned, she described herself as joyful when she found out, and she began preparations for the infant early in the pregnancy. The father was not involved, but Latoya conveyed confidence in her ability as a mother. She believed that an essential part of being a good mother for Crystal included breastfeeding. However, for Latoya, this could not be a simple, straightforward decision.*
>
> *She informed a nurse that she used cocaine and heroin throughout the pregnancy. Latoya described her efforts to "cut down" as much as she could, admitting that she had no immediate plans for abstinence from the drugs. Since drug assay tests were positive for cocaine and heroin in amounts that could damage Crystal, Latoya was told that breastfeeding was not an option for her. She was quite distressed, and insisted that since the drugs had not hurt Crystal during the pregnancy, breastfeeding would not be a problem. Latoya stated that the way she fed her was her own decision.*

Health care providers and the legal system do not agree with Latoya. Additionally, despite strong legal opinions voiced concerning perinatal substance abuse, the written law is unclear and inconsistent. Court-ruled action prohibiting lactation in such situations has so far proven ineffective because enforcement is impossible (Lloyd, 1986). Child-welfare laws in many states do not declare that drug ingestion by the mother even during pregnancy is punishable as child abuse. Consequently, there are few legal precedents in the case of illicit drugs in breast milk.

The situation involving Latoya and Crystal is not uncommon in maternal-child health care. Although substance abuse is not related to socioeconomic status, it is found more frequently in indigent populations who deliver in public institutions, wherein drug histories and testing are done routinely (Vezeau, 1990). Clinicians understand that it is a priority to vigorously support parenting in such scenarios since the mother is often monitored at home by county nursing or social services, unless or until remarkable abuse or neglect is confirmed (Finnegan, 1990).

The examination of divergent approaches to caring will shed light on two points. First, although the concept of caring can help to direct ethical decision making, clinicians must be aware that there are varying interpretations of caring. Second, interventions following from divergent caring approaches are likewise incomparable, and these actions have irrevocable consequences.

NEL NODDINGS' APPROACH TO CARING

Noddings' (1984) definition of caring is based in receptivity. The one who is caring "feels with" the other. In Noddings' words, the one caring "receives the other" totally. This involves feeling, motivational shift, and engrossment with the other. The situation of caring is not an abstract consideration. It is concrete and tied to a real situation. The value emphasized in this paradigm is *in relation*, and in *remaining related.*

Noddings clearly states her ideas regarding rules. Devotion to rules violates the contextual nature of caring. Noddings would prefer a collaboration between those ruled and the rule enforcers in order to keep rules at a minimum, and to interpret rules in light of individual contexts.

For Noddings, mothering and caring are deeply integrated and provide perhaps the best example of caring extant. Mothers feel with their infants naturally and without deliberation. In a particular situation mothers do not initially analyze and interpret, but respond to the feeling content within the interaction. As caring here is based in relationship, any decisions are contextually derived.

Noddings holds that in order to learn how to care one must first be cared for. The future of maintaining the caring attitude is dependent on past and present experiences of caring. Children learn how to care by being cared for themselves. Mothers also learn to care for their infants as they are cared for. It is essential to care for mothers so that they can care for their infants.

Methods of Knowing

Methods of knowing in Noddings' paradigm are grounded in the caring attitude. One is informed not by rules, principles, or even one's own interpretation of a situation, but by being in relationship with the other. By receiving the other, the knower feels with the other, prior to analysis. Knowledge is essentially collaborative.

In the scenario involving Latoya and Crystal, the care provider would need to listen carefully to Latoya, and to be open to the feeling content shared. In this way the clinician would understand the love Latoya held for Crystal and the necessity she felt to breast-feed. Latoya felt joy, but also ambivalence toward Crystal. She believed that breastfeeding would develop her ability to love her child, and that Crystal would feel the connection and not the ambivalence.

In Noddings' paradigm, the clinician would be called to "receive" Crystal also. In spending time with the infant, the clinician would attempt to know what the infant is feeling, what is of value to her and whether breastfeeding matters to her. Some clinicians who work with infants develop an active openness that both invites and listens for communications. Infants effectively share preferences in both audible and nonverbal ways. In this situation, the clinician is obliged to seek cues that could indicate Crystal's feeling about her mother and breastfeeding.

Choices among Options

The basis for choosing from a number of possibilities involves careful consideration of what will best maintain relationships. Although there are many relationships in this situation, the three most germane to my purpose are Latoya to Crystal, Crystal to Latoya, and health care providers to Latoya. Of course, the relationship between the care providers and Crystal would be secondary to their relationship with Latoya, since Latoya has the closest and most obligate position to Crystal. Clinicians would best care for Crystal by supporting Latoya's relationship to Crystal.

Latoya sincerely believed that her relationship to Crystal was dependent on breastfeeding, and thus bottle feeding was not an option. Abstinence from drugs also was not an immediate option. She had tried drug rehabilitation in the past and felt it to be demeaning. When she did find a program during her pregnancy that was acceptable to her, Medicaid would not cover the additional expense. For Latoya, breastfeeding was the only option, and if the desired rehabilitation program could be funded, she would have been agreeable to it.

Crystal molded well into Latoya's arms and gave clear cues about the care she desired. Crystal had great difficulties with controlling the flow of formula from a bottle nipple, and her body was most relaxed during breastfeeding. Nonnutritive sucking was her favorite pastime when awake. Crystal clearly preferred breastfeeding, but could learn to bottle feed.

Latoya expressed her feelings about past relationships with care providers, and none of them were positive. She perceived care providers as "not listening," not caring about her as "someone different from the next guy," and as "vomiting rules about the most stupid things." She did not see care providers as caring, helpful, or as resources in raising her child. Her past experiences had already sabotaged the potential for positive future relationships with care providers.

Noddings, of course, would value the importance of assisting a mother to care for her infant. Of the three relationships described, Noddings also would consider the relationship of Latoya to Crystal as primary. The reciprocal relationship between Latoya and Crystal would benefit Latoya in seeing her efforts and feelings received.

Clinicians well know the dangers in the present foster care situation. However, I believed that if Latoya could maintain a relationship with a care provider she trusted, Crystal would fare no worse in her own mother's hands than in the hands, for example, of a foster parent. In looking at the situation one generation into the future, Crystal would benefit greatly from being cared for consistently by the same person. Although most foster care situations offer an element of physical safety, they do not offer the element of the caring parent.

Forms for Action

In Noddings' (1989) idea of caring, the caring relationship is a good in itself, the good by which other goods are measured. The caring relationship has intrinsic, not instrumental, value. To be caring in Noddings' terms, the clinician would endeavor to maintain that good as end in itself both for Latoya and Crystal. Because a good such as physical safety is simply a means to other ends, it remains a lesser goal.

Caring would involve whatever actions were necessary to maintain relationships—between Latoya and Crystal, Crystal and Latoya, and Latoya and care providers. Action that involved caring would allow for breastfeeding of Crystal in order to maintain connection, and it also would necessitate designation of funds to assist drug rehabilitation in a program that Latoya felt would work. A care provider would maintain close contact with Latoya to check compliance with the drug program in order to validate the safety of breastfeeding. The care provider could observe Crystal physically and could be open to helping Latoya on a variety of levels, working to prevent the real and threatening potential for stress and increased drug usage. There do exist maternal drug rehabilitation programs that can provide home visits by a primary nurse, individual and group counselling, and assay labs to detect drugs in urine and breast milk.

Enactment of such a program would involve commitment of funds from the county. It also would imply trust in Latoya by the county and her care providers. In effect, the county would be acknowledging the importance to maintain the parenting and provider relationships so much desired by Latoya. However, this action plan is fallible and involves risk to all parties concerned, most particularly to Crystal. In Noddings' idea of caring, there can be neither certainty nor uncertainty in a caring relationship. Acceptance of unknown outcomes is at the crux of Noddings' interpretation of caring.

AUDUBON'S APPROACH TO CARING

John James Audubon is known for his love of the natural state of life. I am presenting a literary narrative written by Susan Griffin (1978) that can serve as a powerful example of the positivist approach to caring that is pervasive in the current health care environment.

Because the use of metaphor is uniquely suited to support the complexity and mystery found in the caring situation, both Webster (1990) and Vitz (1990) advocate the use of literary narratives in the discussion of human nature. The following excerpt from Griffin (1978, pp. 113–114) is a work of fiction and a skillfully drawn description of Audubon's way of caring.

> *For weeks upon weeks he observed the habits of this bird. He could create in his mind the posture of the animal as it perched on the highest limb of a magnolia tree. He could predict every movement of the bird; he knew his habits. . . . So the painter did not hurry as he went to find his gun, and he took his time loading it. Then he sequestered himself in weeds about the tree and aimed slowly and carefully. . . . At the sound of the gun the eagle flapped his wings, but could not bear himself into the air and finally fell to the earth. The artist, holding the dying bird in his hands, expressed his wonderment at the expression of the eagle's eye, which at one and the same time blazed as if illuminated with fire, and glazed over with death. As the sun descended the eagle died.*
>
> *Now he was excited. He had a fire built and spent the next hours preparing the bird, stuffing him, mounting him. He had acquired this skill through years of labor and experiment. He used wires to pierce and hold together the body of the bird in the posture he desired, and the result of his efforts created an effect whose grace and naturalness were later said to have rivaled life. . . .*
>
> *Finally he would capture the eagle on paper by placing the body against a background ruled with division lines in squares to correspond to similar divisions on his own paper. And if necessary, in addition, he would measure parts of the bird with a compass. He was meticulous and painted with great accuracy*

*even every barb on every feather, so great was his love for his
subject. And in this, he preserved the birds of America.*

In a clinical situation, we could translate this view to a love of the
"natural" state of things as interpreted by the dominant culture. This
paradigm is not motivated by the value of relationship but by the need
for certainty. What gives rise to caring is a desire to know and to
control in order to promote the "natural" or, more accurately, the
cultural good. Here people are not considered in their individual contexts, rather they are compared to idealized conceptions of what is
"natural," or the normal (cultural) state of affairs. Reciprocity between
the caregiver and the one cared for is not found. In this model of
caring, the care giver is already complete, and does not gain from interaction with the one cared for. The view is detached and normative.

Method of Knowing

The method of knowing in Audubon's paradigm is clear: facts
suffice. Truth obtained from facts is *objective*. Even testimony carrying feeling content is labeled and judged for truthfulness and relevance. In Latoya's situation, the facts were evident: Cocaine and
heroin were found in her urine and in Crystal's. Previous attempts
at drug rehabilitation had failed. Her lifestyle was unstable. She was
without means of support. Although Latoya stated that she loved
her daughter, she did not take the expected steps to indicate her
ability to mother. She did not act as a mother should act. Because
she used drugs, Latoya did not behave in a fashion "natural" to the
dominant culture's view of caring for her daughter in utero.

Choices among Options

In this situation, options for resolution would be limited to those
that society could validate. Because Latoya could not be trusted.
breastfeeding could not be allowed. If the time came when she did
prove to be a "natural" mother, she could breastfeed with close

monitoring of her drug abstinence. If the delay in breastfeeding worked to terminate Latoya's ability to lactate, this would be unavoidable, but necessary.

The only option would be the prevention of Crystal's access to tainted breast milk. Parenting would not be seen as endangered, since many mothers bottle feed and have no difficulties relating to their infants. In addition, if babies are hungry enough, they bottle feed.

Because the drug rehabilitation program serving indigent women was found to be acceptable by the county, extra funds would not be given for a special rehabilitation program found acceptable by Latoya. Decisions among possible options would be made in the interest of Crystal, from the viewpoint of society.

Form for Action

The form for action in Audubon's paradigm would be the acts that would best facilitate "natural" or normal parenting. In Latoya's case this certainly would mean bottle feeding, even if that was not her desire. Latoya would be monitored closely with weekly urine tests at the county drug rehabilitation center, which at present does not provide individual counselling or day care during group sessions. The county nurse would make unannounced visits monthly to evaluate the home environment. If Latoya could prove herself a fit mother according to the plan set by the county, she would then be able to breastfeed and, eventually, she would no longer require monitoring. Any noncompliance with the plan would necessitate forfeiture of Crystal to the county. Certainty is the gold standard for action in Audubon's caring paradigm. This is in contrast to Noddings' approach to caring wherein there is neither surety nor a standard.

DISCUSSION

The caring paradigms of Noddings and Audubon do not consider the case of Latoya and Crystal from the same understanding of caring. Noddings' is a contextual approach in which this situation would be unique. The ways of knowing, the basis for choosing options, and the form for action would all be aimed at the preservation of the primary relationship between Latoya and Crystal. Caring would involve close connection, commitment of resources, and trust toward Latoya.

Caring within Audubon's paradigm would be the same to any mother wanting to breastfeed while ingesting drugs. The physical preservation of Crystal would be of paramount concern, even at the expense of the relationship with her mother. The final word on how to care comes externally from authority figures who do not weigh feelings as heavily as factual information.

At first, it might seem that caring in this paradigm entails the avoidance of risk. In actuality, this interpretation of caring risks everything in order to preserve "normal" physical existence of the young.

The reader may rightly ask where I, as author, stand in this situation. Since I was the nurse here, I cannot take an outsider's viewpoint.

I know that women such as Latoya, often referred to as "drug moms," are decontextualized by principled ethics found in our present system. By not seeing Latoya and Crystal as unique, the issue of caring gains a generic character and obscures the deeper issues at stake.

Nel Noddings (1989), consistent with her book, *Women and Evil,* might say that perinatal substance abuse is society's failure. In locating the fault solely in the mother, this becomes a projection of the evil in society onto women. Noddings defines evil as that which causes pain, separation (loss of connection), and helplessness. Surely, then, in these terms, the situation of Latoya and Crystal qualifies as evil.

Fathers, usually complicit partners in perinatal substance abuse, are not jailed; drug pushers and pimps, most often men, are rarely jailed. Women who attempt healthcare for themselves and their infants frequently are jailed, however. Decisions made regarding Latoya and Crystal were not equitable or caring. They were not determined by respect for connection or attempts toward solution. The decisions were only retribution against a bad mother, and, some thought, an evil woman.

The crux of this issue lies here: Latoya disallowed reasoned and generic approaches because she felt her body was an integral part of herself and her relation with her child. However, she was inconsistent in her ability to act out her beliefs. She appeared unreasonable and inflexible in her relation to her infant as she defined it.

Latoya and Crystal threaten each of us personally. If, as care givers, we remain fully engaged to preserve the relationship, we cannot not maintain a thoroughly objective stance. We are led to a personal assessment of our own morality. Latoya and Crystal compel us to consider the following questions:

Who am I?
What would I do?
Would I do this to my child or to other loved ones?
Have I ever done this?

The answer is, of course, I have, but I have not acknowledged it. I have not recognized the evil in myself, the ability I have to cause pain, break human connection, and cause others to feel helpless. As Nel Noddings (1989) explains, it is essential to understand our own disposition to evil. I might add here that this must happen in order for any action to be caring in addressing this concern for women and children.

The two caring approaches of Noddings and of Audubon are not a dialectic, and they are not polar opposites. It is clear that caring has variant meanings that are currently operating in the practice setting. This is where perinatal substance abuse is not theoretical discussion but involves actions that have irrevocable consequences. Caring often is seen in mandated acts that sever existing and potential human connections.

This story of Latoya and Crystal is not a story of right or wrong. It is a story to listen to and live through, and, as reader, come to your own understandings. You are here not to judge but to live in the story, to be challenged, and to allow for change. As care providers, we cannot subdue societal evil by forcibly trying to eradicate it, but by personally acknowledging it and living with it.

There is an epilogue to this story. Before I present it, I want to share the comments of a journal editor on this paper. She said that not to come either to a synthesis position or to argue for one or the other positions left the discussion too open-ended, too painful. Little did she know that I considered this response the highest praise. I answered her concern by saying that I hope the discussion of caring is not diluted by a debate team style of discussion. This paper is purposefully open-ended, so as not to prescribe the position of the reader.

The problem of perinatal substance abuse exists in its present condition, in part, because of this lack of personal reflection and the desire for pat answers. There is not *a best* approach, only alternatives to the present attempts to address this situation. It *is* a painful situation, fraught with ambiguity, and when I lose sight of that, my response ceases to be personal and ethical. My preference is to leave this story as it is, paused, and waiting for the reader's introspection. Scholarship is not salesmanship, but a compelling invitation to live in a human situation with an open and willing heart.

EPILOGUE

Latoya was court ordered into an outpatient drug rehabilitation program. She was not to breastfeed her daughter until four consecutive weekly urine tests were negative for illicit drugs. At three weeks of age, Crystal was brought into the emergency room in severe hypoglycemia and electrolyte imbalance. Traces of opiates were found in the infant's urine. It was uncertain if drug ingestion or neglect were the root cause of Crystal's illness. Plans were finalized by the county for foster care placement.

The night prior to discharge, Crystal was found missing from her hospital bed. The whereabouts of Crystal and Latoya are, at this time, unknown.

REFERENCES

Benner, P., & Wrubel, J. (1989). *The primacy of caring.* Menlo Park, CA: Addison-Wesley.

Finnegan, L. (1990). *Special currents: Maternal addiction.* Philadelphia: Ross Laboratories Publication.

Griffin, S. (1978). *Woman and nature: The roaring inside her.* New York: Harper & Row.

Koop, C. (1990). *Special currents: Maternal addiction.* Philadelphia: Ross Laboratories Publications.

Lloyd, D. (1986). *Emerging medical-legal issues in child advocacy.* Paper presented at the National Bar Association National Child Advocacy Conference, Chicago, Illinois, November 13–15.

Noddings, N. (1984). *Caring: A feminine approach to ethics and moral education.* Berkeley: University of California Press.

Noddings, N. (1989) *Women and evil.* Berkeley: University of California Press.

Vezeau, T. (1990). *Prevalence of drug use in an urban antepartum population.* Unpublished paper.

Vezeau, T., & Schroeder, C. (1991). Caring approaches: A critical examination of origin, balance of power, embodiment, time and space, and intended outcome. In P. Chinn (Ed.), *Anthology of caring.* New York: National League of Nursing.

Vitz, P. (1990). The use of stories in moral development: New psychological reasons for an old educational method. *American Psychologist, 45*(6), 709–720.

Watson, J. (1985). *Nursing: Human science and human care: A theory of nursing.* Norwalk, CT: Appleton-Century-Croft.

Webster, G. (1990). Nursing and the philosophy of science. In McCloskey, J. & Grace, G. (Eds.), *Current issues in nursing* (3rd ed.). St. Louis: C. V. Mosby.

12

Caring: Being Manifested as Ordinariness in Nursing

Beverley J. Taylor

In this paper, I will explore caring as Being as manifested in ordinariness in nursing, by sharing insights into a phenomenological research project. Here, caring is understood as a humanistic activity (Paterson & Zderad, 1976) lived as an expression of Being (Heidegger, 1962). In addition, I will suggest that human caring, as the essence of nursing, is expressed as a form of moderated love (Campbell, 1984) that creates possibilities of therapeutic relationships between nurses and clients (Pearson, 1988a). Because the present study was still in progress at the time of this writing, and much had yet to be made manifest about the nature of ordinariness in nursing as the research process unfolded, I can offer only an incomplete picture of the entire study.

INTRODUCTION TO THE STUDY

The phenomenological method allows researchers to interpret lived experience as a totality. In this paper, I explored the phenomenon of ordinariness with nurses and patients in a Professorial Nursing Unit (PNU) in Australia. Here, as a basic research premise, human caring is perceived a state of Being through which people express their connectedness to one another in everyday ways befitting their relationships. In a world inhabited by ordinary people, caring as Being is thus manifested as ordinariness in nursing.

The Background of the Study

The term *ordinariness in nursing* was first coined by Alan Pearson (1988b), professor of nursing, who in conversations with colleagues, shared his ideas about the inherent nature of nursing. Pearson said that he felt there was something essentially ordinary in the most effective nursing exchanges, some elusive thing about nurses and nursing, which made extraordinary experiences associated with illness ordinary and manageable for patients. In his own nursing practice, he had made this clinical observation. When he joked and generally took time to interact on an ordinary level with patients, the experience of nursing was enhanced for his patients and for himself.

Taylor (1988) also found that when she asked women in a postnatal ward to describe the midwives who were most effective in caring for them, they described midwives who were "just themselves." The mothers actually differentiated between those midwives who they perceived as "professional in a detached sort of way" and those midwives who were ordinary people as part of their clinical effectiveness. The mothers expressed a preference for the midwives who were "just themselves." The researcher also noticed changes in nursing literature in the ways nurses described nursing. Nursing authors acknowledged the human presence and process in nursing, turning away from previous definitions that had traditionally expressed an instrumental approach to the *products* of nursing care, to language that reflected the *process* of human interactions on a daily level. For example, Paterson and Zderad (1976) conceptualised nursing as "a lived act, a response to a human situation" (p. 19) and explored nursing itself from a phenomenological perspective as "the act of nursing, the intersubjective transactional relation, the dialogue experience, lived in concert between persons where comfort and nurturance prod mutual unfolding" (1978, p. 51).

The background to the present study, therefore, included an interest in the phenomenon of nursing springing from the original idea as expressed by Alan Pearson, the results of the researcher's own work and clinical experience, and the influence of a growing body of nursing literature (Benner, 1983, 1984, 1985; Benner & Wrubel, 1988; Brown, 1986; Chinn & Jacobs, 1987; Fawcett, 1984; Fitzpatrick & Whall, 1989; Leininger, 1985; Marriner-Tomey, 1989; Meleis, 1985; Levine, 1973; McMahon & Pearson, 1991; Moccia, 1986; Paterson, 1971, 1978; Paterson & Zderad, 1976; Travelbee, 1971; Morse, 1989; Oiler, 1982, 1986; Omery, 1983; Parse, 1981, 1985, 1987; Pearson, 1988a,b; Pearson & Vaughan, 1986; Peplau, 1952; Riehl & Roy, 1980; Rieman, 1986; Torres, 1986; Travelbee, 1966, 1971; Watson, 1985; Wiedenbach, 1964) attesting to the everyday nature of nursing as a human activity.

Research questions for this study were inspired by experiencing patients and nurses as ordinary people. I began to wonder about the levels on which patients' and nurses' ordinary humanness interact in a nursing context, with specific interest in the effects of such interactions and what those interactions might reveal about the nature of people as well as the nature of nursing. Above all, I wondered whether it was possible that nurses somehow make ordinary those extraordinary phenomena people encounter in their illness. As such, this exploration of the phenomenon of ordinariness in nursing, attempted to illuminate the nature and effect of ordinariness, discover whether ordinariness enhances the nursing encounter, and draw out meanings and relationships between ordinariness and professionalism in nursing.

THE NATURE OF THE STUDY

Davis (in Norris, 1982) has advanced phenomenological methodology as "an interpretive way of knowing." In this light, phenomenology is a type of qualitative methodology that enables the researcher to "understand empirical matters from the perspective of those being studied" (p. 40). Generated as a consequence of growing disillusionment with empirico-analytical ways of knowing as the only means to reflect the everyday realities of the human condition, phenomenological methodology has developed as a paradigm reflective of "pragmatic activity, that is, everyday understanding and practices, and the study of relational issues, [which] are distinctly different from the study of objects, as in the natural sciences . . ." (Allen, Benner, & Diekelmann, 1986, p. 28).

Nursing and phenomenological methodology share the beliefs and values that people are whole and that they create their own particular meanings. According to Omery (1983), both "consider all that is available in the experience under study, both subjective and objective, and strive to understand the total meaning that the experience has had for the participants (p. 62).

The researcher worked as a participant observer with six registered nurses in a professorial nursing unit. As part of his or her usual nursing care activities, each nurse interacted with four patients, who consented to be part of the research. Following each interaction, the researcher wrote her impressions in a personal-professional journal and audiotaped conversations with the respective nurses and patients to gain their impressions.

Using a theoretical framework of the phenomenological concepts of lived experience (Heidegger, 1962; Husserl, 1965, 1970, 1980), and Dasein (Heidegger, 1962), being-in-the-world (Dreyfus, 1991; Heidegger, 1962), and fusion of horizons (Gadamer, 1976a,b) as an underpinning methodology, the researcher will make an initial hermeneutical analysis and interpretation of the participants' impressions. To provide background to such a discussion, however, a brief review of extant literature follows.

LITERATURE REVIEW

Ordinariness in Nursing

The Oxford Dictionary (multivolume edition) gives the historical meanings of *ordinary* (there is no record of the word *ordinariness*).

In relation to language, *ordinary* is "the most commonly found or attested," and in relation to people, it is "typical of a particular group, average . . ." From these meanings it may be deduced that whatever the unique characteristics of each individual, we as people are bonded by our typically ordinary status of humanity, bearing with it certain qualities that are grouped as average yet are vital for the ways in which we communicate with one another and make meaning of our Being together.

Accounts have been given by nurses and patients of being ordinary in nursing. Gino (1985, p. 30) described her freedom to be herself as a nurse interacting with other human beings:

> *It was the one place I could be totally me. The place I could be as smart, as kind, as giving, and as real as I was capable of being. My patients and I had an understanding past words; we needed each other; we healed each other; and neither of us judged the other. There was no mask, no preference, we were just human beings who because of circumstances had to learn to trust each other and so were allowed to really touch each other.*

Helman (1986) told the story of the illness of her husband, a cancer surgeon, who died of cancer. He recorded on audiotapes his reactions to his dying. He emphasized the need for basic confidence, a sense of hope, concern, compassion, and humility from the people around him; all of which seem to be fairly ordinary human qualities.

The ways nurses and patients experience the nurse–patient relationship are inextricably bound to the humanness of the people involved in caring in nursing. Speaking at a nurse graduation ceremony Pearson (1988) stated:

> *Although I passionately believe that nursing, and, therefore, helping must draw on knowledge, understandings, and insights which are part of good quality professional education, I also believe that it is important to marry this with the ordinariness of being a human being. . . . Most of us are engaged in the process of helping people every day, often without any conscious awareness of "being helpful." The foundation of genuine helping lies in being ordinary. Nothing special. We can offer ourselves, neither more nor less, to*

*others—we have in fact nothing else to give. Anything more is
conceit, anything less is robbing those in distress.*

Phenomenological Perspectives of Caring

In itself, phenomenological perspectives of caring include notions
of being, knowing, nursing, and professionalism. It does so because a
phenomenological perspective of caring perceives nursing as humanistic activity (Paterson & Zderad, 1976) lived as an expression of Being
(Heidegger, 1959, 1962). As the essence of nursing, human caring is
expressed as a form of moderated love (Campbell, 1984) that creates
possibilities of therapeutic relationships between nurses and clients
(Pearson, 1988a,b).

Nursing as Humanistic Activity.   A review of some writing by
Paterson and Zderad (1976), Peplau (1952), and Travelbee (1966) reflects similar humanistic descriptions of nursing, person, health, and
environment. The writing of these scholars will be reviewed here as
early contributions to nursing literature that uses, in each case, an
interpretive approach to attest to the processes involved in everyday
human interaction, thereby departing from the tradition that had
hitherto defined nursing chiefly in terms of products of care.

In relation to nursing, these scholars emphasised interpersonal
relationships and viewed nursing as an interactive process in which
the participants make meaning for themselves. Paterson and Zderad
(1976) conceptualized nursing as "a lived act, a response to a human
situation" (p. 19); Peplau (1952) conceptualized nursing as "being
able to understand one's own behavior to help others identify felt
difficulties" (p. xiii); and Travelbee (1966) focused on the interpersonal process in nursing.

In these views, people are respected for their uniqueness as they
offer to the nurse–patient relationship those understandings about
themselves and others that will optimize the choices of all in the
nursing encounter. Paterson and Zderad (1976) viewed person as an
embodied individual, who is always changing in relation to other
people and things in a temporospatial world. Similarly, for Peplau,
(1952) person was defined in terms of "[people]; an organism liv[ing]

in an unstable equilibrium" (p. 82). Travelbee (1971) described person as "a unique irreplaceable individual, a one-time-being in this world" (p. 26).

Here, health is conceptualisation as a proactive, personally-oriented process through which the individual achieves a sense of spiritual and biopsychosocial integrity. Although Paterson and Zderad (1976) provided no definition of health as such, they wrote that health has also to do with "well-being and more-being" (p. 12). Peplau (1952) defined health as "a word symbol that implies forward movement of personality and other ongoing human processes in the direction of creative, constructive, productive, personal, and community living" (p. 12) whilst Travelbee (1966) agreed that health can be defined by subjective and objective criteria.

From these combined perspectives, environment constitutes a unique sense of self as experienced within and outside the individual. Paterson and Zderad (1976) perceived that people inhabit an inner, biased world as well as an outer, objective world. For Peplau (1952, p. 14), environment was defined in terms of "existing forces outside the organism and in the context of culture" (p. 14). Although Travelbee (1966) did not define environment explicitly, Travelbee did describe human conditions such as pain, hope, and suffering that can be equated with environment.

Nursing, therefore, as humanistic activity, focuses on people interacting in day-to-day encounters, and values nurses and patients for their essential human qualities and potential. Such a view encourages personal growth and personalized approaches to coping with the changes inherent in the experience of illness. Being human is expressed as the person's unique reality as a participant in day to day life.

In Relation to Living as an Expression of Being.   Martin Heidegger (1967) spent most of his life seeking a concrete explanation for the question framed by Aristotle so long ago: "What is being?" and presented an incomplete account of this in his work, *Being and Time*:

For Heidegger, the logos of phenomenology would "make manifest" the way the things themselves (as phenomena) "showed themselves" to be, that is by a process of disclosing or uncovering, thus determining the basic sense of the truth (aletheia) to be the unconcealment by which all beings show themselves to be. The

question of Being . . . required an investigation into the mean-
ing of Time. Heidegger called the being of this questioner who
already had some understanding of Being in general "existence"
Dasein. . . . By using a temporal analysis he attempts to de-
scribe the whole of Dasein, conceived as care, from beginning
(birth) to end (death). (Krell, 1977, pp. 18–20)

In effect, Heidegger suggested that a person is a self-interpreting being who comes to be defined by living a life. People can grasp meaning directly by virtue of their being-in-the-world and embodied intelligence. Notwithstanding the importance of reflective thought, Heidegger was concerned with "the meaning of being," wherein people understand their worlds in terms of the meanings within them.

In nursing, Being is the nurse–patient relationship as it is lived in a particular health care context. The meaning of nursing, then, is embodied by nurses and patients and manifested by them as they interact together. It is that in uncovering some of the nature of Being in nursing that nursing will show itself as it *is*.

Human Caring Expressed as Moderated Love.   Campbell (1984) described nursing as skilled companionship that entails sharing freely and not imposing, thus allowing others to make their own life journey. He conceptualized nursing as involving a bodily presence, in sensing need and accommodating idiosyncracies (sensitivity); in helping onwards to recovery or death (encouraging); in risking to be with, staying with the difficult point (being with); and in allowing the other to go on alone (limitation). Thus, Campbell saw nursing as a situation involving love and companionship. It is possible that the nurse-patient relationship embodies the secrets of the nature of nursing and that caring creates the possibilities of relationships which are therapeutic for the nurse and patient alike.

Therapeutic Relationships between Nurses and Clients.   The word *therapeutic* is derived from the Greek *therapeutikos*, meaning to nurse, serve or cure (Webster, 1972). Therapeutics has taken on a disease-curing connotation, leaving curing to doctors and caring to nurses. The claim has been made, however, that nursing is both carative and curative (Benner & Wrubel, 1988; Kitson, 1984; Pearson, 1988a,b) and that care is the essence of nursing (Watson, 1985; Leininger, 1985). Although caring is the most obvious and regularly described attribute of nursing, these authors argue that it is not the sole mission of nursing. The therapeutic potential of nursing is related to the science of nursing and to the artistry with which nursing care is given.

Exploration of therapeutic approaches in nursing care can get at the heart of practice—the nurse–patient relationship—when professional detachment is abandoned in favor of "closeness between nurse and patient, the idea of partnership, and the development of empathy in nursing" (Pearson, 1988a, p. 12). The effect of this closeness can be healing in nature, a form of therapeutic nursing, no less.

Meutzel (in Pearson, 1988a, p. 89) supported the contention that nursing is a "therapy in itself," confirming the belief that "the power of nursing to promote healing lies . . . in this therapeutic relationship," that endorses "the therapeutic use of self" and the nurse-patient relationship characterized by partnership, intimacy, and reciprocity. These qualities all stand in stark contrast to the professional ethic of distancing and aloofness, whenever professionals avoid the risks of personal involvement by hiding in their "character armor" and acting out a repertoire of behaviors consistent with the "professional manner" (Jourard, 1971).

The Loss of Essential Ordinariness.   Jourard (1971, p. 182) claimed that "people squelch their real selves because they have learned to fear the consequences of authentic being." Jourard was particularly suspicious of the "nurse's bedside manner" as a facade to shield the nurse from the vulnerability inherent in his or her own humanness. He concluded that a nurse who was unwilling to be authentic in self-disclosures was in fact blocking the patient's chances for self-disclosure and authenticity.

It may be possible that, in becoming sophisticated in nursing skills and knowledge, nurses may have lost sight of their essential nature as people. According to Moore (1986), "One of the difficulties with being sophisticated is a negation of the natural . . . they do not have to be separate" (p. 169). Being human is being ordinary; we laugh and cry, we intellectualize and we become downright irrational. Nurses who retain who they are and how they are in spite of temptations to hide inside their "character armor" (Jourard, 1971) may show that the therapeutic effect of nursing has something to do with the way in which nurses can take extraordinary events in patients' lives and make them ordinary somehow. Notwithstanding the need for knowledge and skills in nursing, a nurse whose caring is manifested through day-to-day ordinariness as a person, becomes one with the people with whom he or she is interacting in day-to-day life.

The Temptation to Hide in a Professional Role. Goffman (1974) likens day-to-day life performances to actors on a stage. He acknowledges the nature of real life interactions by stating: "An action staged in a theatre is a relatively contrived illusion and an admitted one; unlike ordinary life, nothing real or actual can happen to the performed characters . . ." (p. 246). Of course, nursing occurs in social contexts that would "upstage" most theatrical performances. The real drama of nursing calls for *total* absorption in the role. In fact, the lived experience of nursing involves a level of involvement and absorption in the situation, because, as Benner and Wrubel (1988) depict it, "there can be no situationless involvement" (p. 82).

The meanings derived from an exploration of the shared understandings of nurses and patients, as they interact in a health care context, can illuminate the nature of nursing as it is lived by its participants. Such meanings bear relevance to people living in the world of nursing, whose being-in-the-world relates to the temporality of their existence, in showing how "the person is anchored in a present that is made meaningful by past experience and by the person's anticipated future" (Benner & Wrubel, 1988, p. 412).

SHARING SOME OF THE MEANING UNCOVERED

At the time of writing this paper, the final stage of interpretation of study participants' impressions had not been reached. The researcher had enjoyed being a participant observer in the life of the nursing unit, observing nurse–patient interactions, and compiling accounts of her own impressions, as well as those so generously offered to her by the patients and nurses participating in the study. The following accounts of an interaction are offered as an example of what sort of things were showing themselves to *be* in this study. As the impressions are presented, I am reminded of the sense of awe I felt whenever I was taken into other people's worlds in trust and confidence.

To share impressions in the order in which they unfolded, I will present my own account first, then as I talked with the respective patient and nurse. For the purposes of this paper, the following versions have been abbreviated.

Max and Jane

Max was born on February 20, 1949. When he was 13 years old he experienced a cerebral subarachnoid haemorrhage. Four years later, after further neurological sequelae, he began to manifest signs of triplegia. Max lives at home with his mother, who supports him in looking after himself. He spends time in the local hospital whenever he has problems associated with immobility and he visits a large city hospital for assessment and rehabilitation as necessary. He was admitted to the professorial nursing unit on January 23, 1991, to allow healing of a sacral decubitis ulcer. Jane is a Primary Nurse working in the professorial nursing unit (PNU). She cares for Max whenever he is admitted to the nursing unit. Jane invited me to accompany her while she was interacting with Max one morning. She was to assist Max in evacuating his bowel.

Impressions of the Interaction. I (referred to here as *Bev*) recorded her impressions thus:

> *6/2/91. Jane tells me she is ready. We have just returned from morning tea together and she has decided that she will attend to Max now we are back. She talks with me at the desk. She explains the gift box. It was given to her by the nursing staff at a party, because she has a reputation of being "into this sort of stuff." As she begins to open the box, I see some writing on the outside. It looks like a quite usual gift box, but I sense it is not by the way Jane is smiling and going slightly flushed. "I told Max I would present it to him today," she says, as she takes off the lid. Inside is a long coiled piece of plastic faeces on a bed of pink-coloured packing material. I am surprised and I laugh. We both laugh. "Isn't it life like!" I say.*
>
> *We walk together to Max. Another nurse comes alongside, to see the presentation. Max smiles and shifts in the bed. "I won't*

open it now," he says. Jane laughs lightly and leans into him. "Oh
yes you will!" she says. The other nurse agrees with the prompt
and Max sneaks a quick look. He smiles broadly and leans back
not talking as we all enjoy a laugh together. The other nurse
leaves and we are left to get on with the procedure. Max tells Jane
what she will need; extra moisture-resistant "blueys," a plastic
bag, and so on. Although Jane and Max have a long history of
being together in the previous PNU site, Jane has not yet done the
"new way" of bowel evacuation which has been used since Max's
last admission. Jane knows she will be pressing on Max's abdo-
men, whilst he evacuates his own bowel, by anal stimula-
tion. . . . Through the screens the sound of a radio opposite us is
loud and cheerful. We hear Hothouse Flowers sing "I Can See
Clearly Now." . . . I think about the flimsy barrier of the cur-
tain, the "outside" and the "inside" coexisting in a comfortable
sort of way.

The account continues to describe the whole of the procedure,
including a wash and bed tidy, but we will leave it at this point.

Max's Impressions.   6/2/91. We began by talking about his reactions to the "gift box," that involved him going along with the joke,
because he perceived that it was fun. We then talked about the
bowel procedure.

> Bev: What we had to do, I guess to other people, would sound
>   fairly extraordinary, but for you it's a common occur-
>   rence isn't it?
> Max: And for Jane, she's used to it.
> Bev: That's right. So, how does something like that affect you
>   personally?
> Max: It's an everyday situation.
> Bev: Is there anything that you can think of that makes it
>   "everyday," what is it about the way it happens that
>   makes it an everyday situation?
> Max: Neither of us like doing it. We both know what has to be
>   done, so it's not an embarrassment. Neither of us feel
>   embarrassed by what's going on.

The conversation continues and later Max says . . .

Max: *Certain people are well aware that I haven't reached my
maximum potential. I still haven't found out how far I
can go.*

Bev: *And you're just searching for that are you?*

Max: *Yes and no. I'm just trying to retain maximum independence.*

Bev: *Getting back to Jane. Is there any way in which
Jane helps you to do that? assists you to maintain your
independence?*

Max: *Yes. She quietly lets me try my own techniques first before
she intervenes. She would intervene at any time if something went wrong. . .*

The conversation continues, but we will leave it at this point.

Jane's Impressions.   6/2/91. Jane and the researcher began by talking about the "gift box" she presented to Max. The researcher asked
her how it was that she felt okay about sharing the joke with him.

Jane: *Because I think I know him really well, we've got a good
rapport. I like him as a person. We call a spade a spade,
we've had a few run-ins in the first admission.*

Bev: *Raised words?*

Jane: *No, not particularly raised words or raised voices, but just
a matter of, "Hey come on get your act together, stop sort
of feeling sorry for yourself." Like he was feeling very sorry
for himself at the weekend just prior to when I came back
from holidays. But I don't know, we just clicked and that
was it. I can sort of have a joke with him and he can tell
me to shut my face or do whatever and let me know it's not
meant to be offensive or anything. Yet, I also think I know
when it's time to back off.*

Bev: *Can you tell me a bit about that conversation, how it
came about and what happened?*

Jane: *He had actually turned around to me and said he was
really feeling depressed. He'd been swearing at the staff*

and telling them to get lost and didn't want anything done. Now, the first time I went in to see him he was asleep, so I just left him and then when he woke up he had somebody there (visiting). When I saw he was awake the first thing I did was I went over and gave him a kiss on the cheek and a cuddle. I said "I didn't think I'd see you back here again." And his visitor said "Oh, you know someone." I looked at him and he found it very difficult to talk and I thought, "Hey this isn't the Max that I sort of know," so I just let it ride. Later on in the afternoon I went to see him and asked him about his (pressure care) turn. He said, "Oh you do what you like," and I said, "Max, I don't do what I like, I do what you want me to do." "Oh," he said "The others do this that and the other," and I said "Where's the fight gone Max?" He started to cry and the first thing I did was put my arms around him, because I'm a tactile person. I know if people don't want to be touched. He didn't back off. He didn't freeze or anything. He just laid there. He just started and said, "Well you know what drugs I'm on and everything else. I've been on psychiatric drugs for so long, the psychiatrist has written me off." I said, "What a load of crap." I said, "You go out and ask a 100 people out there and I bet there's about 80 or so of them on something to keep them going for the day." I said, "If that's the way you feel, what's the point? You're feeling sorry for yourself that you're having to take them to keep you going through the day." I think I floored him.

Bev: *So what was his reaction?*

Jane: *His reaction was he just sat there. He said, "You're humoring me." I said, "I've never humored you." I said, "We've always called a spade a spade." He wouldn't actually say yes, or no. Then afterwards he turned around and said, "Well, I've got a bit more living to do," and I said, "Good, I'm glad," so I gave him another hug.*

Bev: *How did you feel at that moment?*

Jane: *I felt good, because I was crying as well. The eye contact wasn't there first of all, but when he said, "I've got some*

*living to do," he looked straight at me and I felt Oh! I said,
"Wasn't this the real Max that we saw the first time?" He
said, "No, you wouldn't like the real Max." And I said,
"Why?" He said, "Because I'd be in the looney bin," and I
said, "Well you'd be in good company then wouldn't you."
He looked at me. I said, "We'd all be over there with you."
I said, "Because we all hide a certain amount of ourselves
and we just put over what we want to put over to people."
Since then he's been laughing and joking and the snide
remarks are back again. He's a nice guy, he puts himself
down just too much, he's an intelligent guy. I can see the
frustration in him. He's been incapsulated in this body
that just won't do things for him, he's really quite frustrated. I like him as a person.*

Later, I sat quietly and thought about Max and Jane and wrote
these words:

> *He is tired of the sentence,*
> *Years of life without walking,*
> *He is tired of the people*
> *Who stand over his bed.*
> *He feels labelled and cornered*
> *No respite seems likely*
> *From the sounds and words*
> *Moving around in his head.*
>
> *She sees him as a person*
> *She sees him as young*
> *With potential and intelligence*
> *Promise and hope.*
> *Her words are of challenge*
> *Tempered with kindness*
> *All the courage he needs*
> *She conveys in a joke.*

I invited Jane to look at the accounts of the interaction with Max
so that she could give her impressions of their accuracy. I also
wanted Jane to realize that she is an important part of this paper and

of the research. Jane took the transcript home over night and spoke to me the next day. She said the poem touched her, especially the first line: "He is tired of the sentence." As she related her reactions, she began to cry. She said, "It is Max."

At this stage, given the nature of phenomenological methodology and the unfinished status of the study, it is not appropriate to attempt an analysis of the interaction. However, the discoveries shared in the literature review of what has been written about the nature of the nurse–patient relationship may make it possible for the reader to make some interesting inferences in this abbreviated account of the interaction.

CONCLUSION

In this paper, I've held the premise that nurses, whose caring is manifested through ordinariness, optimise the chances of "right action" in therapeutic interpersonal relationships, making the phenomena of illness commonplace and somehow manageable for people who find themselves in need of nursing care. In the phenomenological perspective used here, I have taken nursing caring as a humanistic activity (Paterson & Zderad, 1976) lived as an expression of being (Heidegger, 1962). In addition, as the essence of nursing, human caring is expressed as a form of moderated love (Campbell, 1984) that creates possibilities of therapeutic relationships between nurses and clients (Pearson, 1988a,b). I have suggested that nurses may be tempted to hide in their professional roles, thereby diminishing the value of their essential ordinariness as humans in the nursing encounter.

Although I have yet to share the composition and message of the finished research, I hope this presentation reveals that people's intersubjective realities are vibrant and hold the promise of combining in striking ways.

In closing, I will share a wonderful quote of the philosopher-mathematician, Moritz Geiger, concerning the "psychological" function of art, I discovered while reading Spiegelberg's (1976) historical account of the phenomenological movement:

Isn't it strange? Here we have uninteresting people such as one can meet everyday. . . , whose nondescript physiognomies we pass by without paying any attention: Along comes Rembrandt and depicts them in all their plainness —and now we stand gripped and delighted before the painting of the Night Watch, and before those commonplace people who shock us in life. . . . How does this happen? What is the nature of the psychical process which achieves such miracles, which produces effects that differ in quality from anything we experience elsewhere, and that can be compared only with being gripped (Ergriffenheit) with religious feeling and metaphysical insight?

It is possible that by returning to the caring nature of the "thing itself" called nursing, we may experience something of the effects of which Geiger speaks. Miracles in nursing happen everyday; they are brought about in quiet, unassuming ways and are manifested in ordinary human qualities and encounters that happen day after day. If we use a phenomenological lens to focus on this humanistic activity, it is possible that we may see the familiar and commonplace in nursing with new eyes and stand in awe of the beauty of its ordinariness. In this way, we can come to know the nature of the "thing itself" and portray the image of its Being as the essential artistry of nursing.

REFERENCES

Allen, D., Benner, P., & Diekelmann, N. L. (1986). Three paradigms for nursing research: Methodological implications. In P. L. Chinn (Ed.), *Nursing research methodology: Issues and implementation*. Rockville, MD: Aspen.

Benner, P. (1983). Uncovering the knowledge embedded in clinical practice. *Image: Journal of Nursing Scholarship, 15*(3), 36–41.

Benner, P. (1985). Quality of life: A phenomenological perspective on explanation, prediction, and understanding in nursing science. *Advances in Nursing Science, 8*(1), 1–14.

Benner, P. (1984). *From novice to expert: Excellence and power in clinical nursing practice*. Menlo Park, CA: Addison-Wesley.

Benner, P., & Wrubel, J. (1988). *The Primacy of caring. Stress and coping in health and illness.* Menlo Park, CA: Addison-Wesley.

Brown, L. (1986). The experience of care: Patient perspectives. *Topics in Clinical Nursing, 8*(2), 56–62.

Campbell, A. V. (1984). *Moderated love. A theology of professional care.* Bristol: Photobooks.

Chinn, P. L., & Jacobs, M. K. (1987). *Theory and nursing: A systematic approach.* St. Louis: C. V. Mosby.

Dreyfus, H. L. (1991). *Being-in-the-world: A commentary on Heidegger's being and time.* Cambridge: MIT Press.

Gadamer, H-G. (1976a). *Truth and method.* G. Barden & J. Cumming (Eds. & Trans.). New York: Seabury.

Gadamer, H-G. (1976b). The universality of the hermeneutical problem. In D. E. Linge (Trans.), *Philosophical hermeneutics.* Berkeley: University of California Press.

Gino, C. (1985). *Rusty. A true story.* London: Pan Books.

Goffman, E. (1974). *The presentation of self in everyday life.* London: Pelican Books.

Fawcett, J. (1984). *Analysis and evaluation of conceptual models of nursing.* Philadelphia: F. A. Davis.

Fitzpatrick, J. J., & Whall, A. L. (1989). *Conceptual models of nursing: Analysis and application.* Norwalk, CT: Appleton and Lange.

Heidegger, M. (1959). *Introduction to metaphysics* (R. Manheim, Trans.). New Haven, CT: Yale University Press.

Heidegger, M. (1962). *Being and time.* (J. Macquarie & E. Robinson, Trans.). New York: Harper & Row.

Helman, E. (1986). *An autumn life. How a surgeon faced his fatal illness.* London: Faber and Faber.

Husserl, E. (1965). *Phenomenology and the crisis of philosophy.* (Q. Lauer, Trans.). New York: Harper & Row.

Husserl, E. (1970). *The Crisis of the European sciences and transcendental phenomenology.* Evanston, IL: Northwestern University Press.

Husserl, E. (1980). *Phenomenology and the foundations of the sciences* (T. E. Klein & W. E. Pohl, Trans.). The Hague: Martinus Nijhoff Publishers.

Jourard, S. M. (1971). *The transparent self.* New York: Van Nostrand.

Kitson, A. L. (1984). *Steps towards the identification and development of nursing therapeutic functions in the care of hospitalised elderly.* (Unpublished doctoral thesis). Coleraine: University of Ulster.

Krell, D. F. (1977). *Martin Heidegger: Basic writings.* New York: Harper & Row.

Leininger, M. M. (1985). *Qualitative research methods in nursing.* Orlando, FL: Grune and Stratton.

Levine, M. E. (1973). *Introduction to clinical nursing.* Philadelphia: F. A. Davis.

Marriner-Tomey, A. (Ed.) (1989). *Nursing theorists and their work.* St. Louis: C. V. Mosby.

McMahon, R., & Pearson, A. (Eds) (1991). *Nursing as therapy.* London: Chapman and Hall.

Meleis, A. I. (1985). *Theoretical nursing: Development and progress.* Philadelphia: Lippincott.

Moccia, P. (Ed.) (1986). Theory development and nursing practice: A synopsis of a study of the theory-practice dialectic. In *New approaches to theory development.* New York: National League for Nursing.

Moore, M.-M. (1986). *Bartholomew: I come as brother.* Taos, NM: High Mesa Press.

Morse, J. M. (Ed.) (1989). *Qualitative nursing research: A contemporary dialogue.* Rockville, MD: Aspen.

Norris, C. M. (1982). Concept clarification: Evolving methods in nursing. In *Concept clarification in nursing,* Rockville, MD: Aspen, 37–47.

Oiler, C. (1982). The phenomenological approach in nursing research. *Nursing Research, 31*(3), 171–181.

Oiler, C. (1986). Phenomenology: The method. In P. Munhall & C. Oiler (Eds.), *Nursing research: A qualitative perspective.* Norwalk, CT: Appleton-Century-Crofts.

Omery, A. (1983, January). Phenomenology: A method for nursing research. *Advances in Nursing Science,* 49–63.

Oxford English Dictionary (1989). United Kingdom: Oxford Clarendon Press and Oxford University Press.

Parse, R. R. (1981). *Man-living-health: A theory of nursing.* New York: John Wiley & Sons.

Parse, R. R., Coyne, A. B., & Smith, M. S. (1985). *Nursing research: Qualitative methods.* Bowie, MD: Brady.

Parse, R. R. (1987). *Nursing science: Major paradigms, theories and critiques.* Philadelphia: W. B. Saunders.

Paterson, J. (1971, March–April). From a philosophy of clinical nursing to a method of nursology. *Nursing Research, 20*(2), 143–146.

Paterson, J. G. (1978). The tortuous way toward nursing theory. In *Theory development: What, why, how?* New York: National League for Nursing, 49–65.

Paterson, J. G., & Zderad, L. T. (1976). *Humanistic nursing.* New York: John Wiley & Sons.

Pearson, A. (Ed.) (1988a). *Primary nursing.* London: Croom Helm.

Pearson, A. (1988b). Unpublished Lakeside Graduation Address, Ballarat, Victoria.

Pearson, A., & Vaughan, B. (1986). *Nursing models for practice.* London: Heinemann Nursing.

Peplau, H. (1952). *Interpersonal relations in nursing: A conceptual frame of reference for psychodynamic nursing.* New York: Putnam's.

Riehl, J. P., & Roy, C. (1980). *Conceptual models for nursing practice.* New York: Appleton-Century-Crofts.

Rieman, D. J. (1986). The essential structure of a caring interaction: Doing phenomenology. In P. Munhall & C. Oiler (Eds.), *Nursing research: A qualitative perspective.* Norwalk, CT: Appleton-Century-Crofts.

Spiegelberg, H. (1976). *The phenomenological movement: A historical introduction.* The Hague: Martinus Nijhoff.

Swaffield, L. (1988, June 8). Communication: Tuned in. *Nursing Times, 84*(23), 28–31.

Taylor, B. (1988). *What are the patients' perceptions of the usefulness of information given to them by nurses and what are the nurses' perceptions of their roles and constraints as teachers in giving effective patient education in a postnatal ward?* A research paper submitted in partial fulfilment of the requirements for the degree of Master of Education, Deakin University, Geelong.

Torres, G. (1986). *Theoretical foundations of nursing.* Norwalk, CT: Appleton-Century-Crofts.

Travelbee, J. (1966). *Interpersonal aspects of nursing.* Philadelphia: F. A. Davis.

Travelbee, J. (1971). *Interpersonal aspects of nursing.* Philadelphia: F. A. Davis.

Watson, J. (1985). *Nursing: Human science and human care. A theory of nursing.* Norwalk, CT: Appleton-Century-Crofts.

Webster, N. (1972). *The international Webster encyclopedic dictionary.* New York: Tabor House.

Wiedenbach, E. (1964). *Clinical nursing: A helping art.* New York: Springer.

13

Nursing: The Caring Practice "Being There"

Katie Eriksson

CARING COMMUNION

Throughout the 1980s and continuing into the 1990s, great consideration has been given to the idea, origins, and essence of caring. The work of Lanara (1981), Leininger (1988), and Watson (1988) is exemplary here. To an ever increasing extent, caring research has been directed toward the search for answers relative to the most basic questions about human caring. Such questions have been raised to lay appropriate foundations, both theoretical and practical, for development of the best possible caring of the human being via qualitative methods.

The goal of a discipline is to get close to the core, the very essence of the actual reality of concern. Caring science is defined through its ontology, what characterizes caring itself. Here, of course, ontology deals with existing entities in a certain reality. In this light, the ontology of caring science concerns itself with five major theses:

1. Man is a whole of body, soul, and spirit.
2. Man is basically a religious human being, but not everyone has personally accepted this dimension.
3. "The value of man," human dignity, is the ability of an individual to shape his or her life and being.
4. Health is more than absence of illness. To be healthy is to be whole, to experience and feel whole as regards body, soul, and spirit. Health is part of life. Health has no meaning unless life has meaning.
5. Caring is naturally human, a manifestation of human love. The core of caring is to "purge" (to clean), play, and learn in a spirit of faith, hope, and love.

I have developed these theses over a span of 20 years (Eriksson, 1981, 1988, 1989). The main research method has been a logical analysis of presuppositions to establish valid principles in nursing or caring science (Nygren, 1972, p. 217).

Motive Research in Caring Science

The discipline comprises systematic caring science and contextual (i.e., applied) caring science. In systematic caring science, research tasks include investigation of basic motives for caring and the introduction of a system of theses founded on such basic motives (Eriksson, 1988, p. 29). The system of theses, as offered, depicts a special inner structure or pattern which is formed according to the basic motives, as well as to certain structural principles. Here motive research investigates what brings about coherence and connects different elements—the cornerstone idea, or the basic motive within a certain science (Nygren, 1972).

Although motive research is similar to research into the history of ideas—the study of complexes of ideas, their origins, structure, development, and organization in society as a whole—there is a difference. In motive research, no emphasis is given to historical-genetic connections.

According to Nygren (1966), "A basic motive gives a certain prejudiced response to a question of the utmost importance, which from the categorical point of view can be considered as a basic question" (p. 23).

The aim of motive research is to find the essential context, the binding of the elements, the leading idea. The idea of motive research applied to caring science is, in an objective way, to show the characteristics of caring. The basic motive for human caring cannot be found in technical or rational biases. Nursing research based on technical paradigms alone has estranged us from the basic motive of caring.

The Basic Motive and the Basic Category. One of the fundamental strivings in caring science is to find basic categories, a focus that is comprehensive and includes the meaning of caring. For instance, could the concepts of "health care" and "care of the sick" be referred to, in the classical sense, the same basic category, or do they have different connotations?

According to Nygren (1972, p. 36), when an individual makes a caring judgement, we can discern by analysis that that individual has applied a caring, rather than a medical or psychological, category. In order to understand the meaning of the judgement, however, we must know what kind of caring criterion is being employed, what fundamental caring motive underlies it, and what caring idea the individual making it favors.

The caring ideal must be distinguished from a concept when we know the fundamental motive which gives it its distinctive character and determines its meaning.

The caritas motive, the idea of caring as an expression of human love and charity, is an idea that has shaped caring for centuries. Unfortunately, there is hardly any other guiding idea that has been so invisible in nursing practice. Suffering is a basic category for all forms of human caring. True caring is not just an abstract thought, a philosophy, or ideology; the performance of caring also is most tangible work, encountering suffering in real situations, a true being there (Eriksson, 1990).

The Caritas Motive

The caritas motive can be traced through semantics, anthropology, and the history of ideas. The concept of "caring" is connected with the concept of "love" through the French word "cherir" (from "cher," in English "dear"). "Cherir" as well as the English word "cherish" (which means to hold dear, feel or show love for) originate from the Latin word "carus" (in English, "care," "caring"), which means love. "Caritas" means human love and charity (Nygren, 1966). Anthropologically, the essence of the human being is love. Giving love is a human characteristic (Lévinas, 1988). The history of ideas states that the foundation of the caring profession through the ages has been an inclination to help and minister to those suffering (Lanara, 1981).

As the basic motive of caring, the caritas motive implies the core, that is, responsibility for the other and caritative caring. In other words, caring is based on human love. However, this does not mean that caring science disregards the fact that technical measures also are necessary in nursing. The core of nursing is caring; the entities being to purge (i.e., to make physically, mentally, and spiritually clean), play, and learn in a spirit of love, truth, and hope (Eriksson, 1987).

Caritative caring means that we take "caritas" into use when caring for the human being in health and suffering. In the professional sense, we use "caritas" for a certain purpose, for the human being who is more or less suffering, or in some kind of distress and need. Caritative caring is a manifestation of the love which "just exists." It has a caring effect through its very existence in a caring culture.

There is caritative caring in nursing practice which is derived from the original idea of human love and charity. In an empirical research study, Eriksson (1990) provides evidence for this statement. Analyzing nurses' written descriptions of what they experienced as being caritative caring situations, Eriksson validated the proposition that the idea of caritas is still implied in caring today. Faith, hope, and love—the basic elements of caring—are conveyed through caring, playing, and learning in both large and small everyday nursing tasks. According to Eriksson, the caring pattern that emerged from the data originated in a felt responsibility for the other, a real interest in the patient. Something of that suggested by Mayerhoff (1971) could be read between the lines.

Caring will become natural with the nurse's focus on the patient when the nurse feels his or her responsibility is to do all he or she can for the patient. Results show that there is a tendency to restrict caritative caring to situations where only patient and nurse are present. Will the nurse's responsibility and focus be directed toward the situation (the medical-technical nursing actions) if another person (e.g., a physician) is present? Nonetheless, it is caritative caring that should point the way to the development of the discipline.

Suffering as a Basic Category of Caring

The alleviation of suffering might be an inherent aspect of all forms of humanistic activity. Adopting suffering as a basic category of caring, however, can be criticized by claiming that it is too inclusive a concept. Yet, the aim here is precisely the opposite: to delimit the general concept of care in order to characterize its various forms and traditions. Eliminating "suffering" and care deprives us of caring, and vice versa: with suffering we acquire a context that does justice to certain caring traditions.

Caring science does not dispute the existence of suffering. Although the ideals of the discipline are soundness and health, suffering is the point at which caring begins. Not until the patient has come to terms with his or her suffering can he or she truly hope for recovery and growth. Being a humanistic discipline, caring science has its roots in all aspects of human life. Modern man fears life and death alike.

Suffering is the deepest, most tacit, and most naked mode of human existence. It differs from pain in that it does not have the same direct language. Although suffering and pain often are present in the same life situation, it can be difficult to define the point at which suffering ends and pain begins.

Current language is not so rich in nuance, and it is no longer natural to use the term "suffering" in speech. This is in fact paradoxical. Only by recognizing suffering can we experience pain and, through compassion, share suffering.

Suffering and Health. Suffering can be explained in many ways, depending on which view is chosen. However, all suffering has one common denominator. If we perceive health as a whole, then one part of health is suffering. Anyone who has not seen the meaning of suffering is in some way unable to hold his or her own as a whole person.

Suffering and health belong together. If suffering is regarded as a natural part of life, then it is part of health. We know that human suffering can, for various reasons, become intolerable for reasons other than our ability to suffer. Through facing suffering we learn to endure it, and the experience becomes a positive resource in life. Unendurable suffering in turn cripples us and prevents us from growing. Health is endurable suffering.

The Alleviation of Suffering. The alleviation of human suffering has at all times been the very heart of all forms of caring. The problems of suffering are associated with the problems of mankind. Suffering means the experience of something that hurts. The problem of suffering is connected with the question of good and evil. Suffering has many faces and has in the course of history undergone a transformation that affects all human phenomena.

An understanding of suffering is fundamental to caring science. We can not reduce suffering to a certain state of being, a social phenomenon, or anything else; we must encounter suffering as suffering.

Suffering is the main, basic category of all caring. Suffering provides caring with its own character and identity. All forms of caring aim in one way or an other to alleviate suffering. We have to admit the fact that many forms of caring have become estranged from the basic category and would hardly recognize it. As a category, suffering also satisfies the demand for communion, in other words, it is one link between contexts. In different contexts of course, suffering and the ways of overcoming it are concerned in different ways (Nygren, 1972).

In summary:

- The basic structure of caring is the relationship between the patient and the nurse.
- The basic category of caring is suffering, that is, suffering is what motivates all kinds of caring.

- The motive for caring to alleviate the patient's suffering is based on the caritas motive.
- Caring communion—true caring—will occur in an unselfish relationship with another.

If the basic assumption is that caring communion is the context of caring, it may be supposed that communion is the source of power and meaning in caring. It is this inner context which is the basis for the inner desire to care.

Caring Communion

According to a lexical definition, communion means "the act of sharing, an intimate relationship with deep understanding" (Webster's New World Dictionary, 3rd ed.). Caring communion, true caring, occurs when the one caring in a spirit of caritas alleviates the suffering of the patient.

According to Buber (1963), May (1983), and Tillich (1952), homo sapiens are born to live in communion with themselves and others. Communion is the basis for all humanity. One logical consequence of this premise is that all forms of caring are variations on human communion.

Joining in communion means creating possibilities for the other. Lévinas (1988) suggests that considering someone as one's own son implies crossing the border of "the possible." In this relationship, the individual perceives the other person's possibilities as if they were his or her own. This requires the ability to shake off the liability of individual identity, something which is just one's own, and move toward something which is no longer just one's own but which belongs to oneself. It is one of the deepest forms of communion. According to Lévinas, it is fatherhood. It is one of the deepest forms of communion.

The Basis of Caring Communion. In all descriptions of caring situations in my empirical research study (Eriksson, 1990), I have included caritative elements. The results support the following basic premise: all true caring communion is based on the caritas motive.

At the heart of caring communion are different prerequisites which appear to be most important for its experience. Heading the list is a genuine, mature, and professional attitude. This is something more than "regular" neighborliness and friendship. The professional attitude implies responsibility, genuineness, courage, and wisdom.

Caring communion requires meeting in time and space, an absolute, lasting presence. As a quantity, time is of no great significance, but the quality of sharing time with somebody is important. This kind of time experience is not objectively connected with time experience in general; it has more to do with the ability for a human experience of presence.

According to my research data, caring arises from a form of emotional ability, an ethical motive, and a willingness to do something special. The ability to minister, to give the whole self, is of the utmost importance in almost all situations.

An open view of science allowing for the unknown, the idiographic, is a necessary prerequisite for the ability to enter into creative action.

Substance and Entities of Caring Communion. The substance of caring communion can be summarized as the art of making something very special out of something less special. Caring communion is a creative act which can imply different forms and contents, but it is characterized by intensity, vitality, openness, and possibilities. The emotional experience within caring communion implies the ability to "cry with those who cry, laugh with those who laugh, grieve with those who grieve, and be happy with those who are happy" (Leininger, 1988).

Caring communion provides a culture that is characterized by warmth, presence, rest, respect, frankness, and tolerance. Fundamental entities are care, eye contact, listening, and language. Caring communion is characterized by fighting together, succeeding, being together, and going through something together. The situations may vary: a struggle for existence or death; sudden, dramatic, even incurable desease; abortion; the simpler actions of washing, or feeding; or occasions of fear, pain, and insomnia. The experience of caring communion does not directly depend on the nature of the situation.

The meaning of caring communion can be summarized as the ability to do good for another person. From the patient's point of view, caring community means the experience of being a subject, of being someone special and important to another person; an experience of someone's responsibility, and willingness to do good for me— an experience of good caring. In the present study, one description of caring revealed this: "She looked like another person, her eyes were clear and she was relaxed . . . and she had courage to live, had to live in spite of the difficult situation." From the nurse's point of view, there is a meaning of being present, the experience of ministering to the patient, giving something of oneself for the purpose of something very important in the actual situation.

True caring is not a form of behaviour, not a feeling or a state. It is an ontology, a way of living. It is not enough to be there, to share— it is *the* way—the spirit in which it is done.

REFERENCES

Buber, M. (1963). *Jag och Du*. Stockholm: Bonniers.

Eriksson, K. (1981). *The patient care process—An approach to curriculum construction within nursing education*. The Development of a Model for the Patient Care Process and an Approach for Curriculum Development Based on the Process of Patient Care. Helsinki: Department of Education, University of Helsinki No. 94.

Eriksson, K. (1987). *Vårdandets idé*. (The idea of caring) Stockholm: Almqvist & Wiksell.

Eriksson, K. (1988). *Caring science as a discipline*. Åbo: Åbo Akademi.

Eriksson, K. (1989). *Hälsans idé*. (The idea of health). Stockholm: Almqvist & Wiksell.

Eriksson, K. (1990). *Pro caritate. Caritative caring—A situational analysis and empirical study concerning the existence of caritative caring*. Åbo: Åbo Akademi.

Lanara, V. (1981). *Heroism as a nursing value*. Athen: Sisterhood Evniki.

Leininger, M. M. (1988). *Care—The essence of nursing and health*. Detroit: Wayne State University Press.

Lévinas, E. (1988). *Etik och oändlighet*. Stockholm-Lund: Symposion Bokförlag och tryckeri AB.

May, R. (1983). *Den omätbara människan: om människosynen i existentialisk psykologi och terapi.* (Margareta Edgardh, Trans.) (original title: The discovery of being: Writings in existential psychology). Stockholm: Bonniers.

Mayerhoff, M. (1971). *On caring.* New York: Harper & Row.

Nygren, A. (1966). *Eros och Agape.* Stockholm: AB Tryckmans.

Nygren, A. (1972). *Meaning and method.* London.

Tillich, P. (1952). *The courage to be.* Yale University Press. (Swedish trans.: Modet att vara till. Stockholm: AB Tryckmans)

Watson, J. (1988). *Nursing: Human science and human care. A Theory of Nursing.* Colorado: Brown and Company.

Webster's New World Dictionary of American English. (3rd ed.) New York: Webster's New World.

14

The Process of Inflicting Pain in Nursing: Caring Relationship or Torture?

Carole Schroeder

In a recent article, Newman, Sime, and Corcoran-Perry (1991) described the focus of the discipline of nursing as the study of caring in the human health experience. Definitions of caring in nursing are diverse, but all involve some form of relationship between nurses and patients. In fact, caring relationships can be broadly grouped into two areas: the nurse–patient relationship as viewed as a means to an end (usually health, healing, transcendence, or growth) or the nurse–patient relationship as viewed as an end in itself, or, as Gadow terms it (in Veazeu & Schroeder, 1991, p. 15), "engagement with no purpose." Amidst these views and more, in nursing there is agreement that a human relationship must exist in some form for caring to occur.

Yet, a disturbing paradox exists in nursing practice: many, if not most, nursing "procedures" require the nurse's participation in acts which inflict pain or cause suffering to another human being. In order not to suffer with the person in pain, nurses frequently disembody, or dissociate, with their own body; in this way, the patient's body becomes an object to be treated, and the nurse does not have to recognize or feel the pain he or she may create. For the person in pain, the experience of feeling pain is one of extreme embodiment; the experience of the nurse is one of extreme disembodiment. The patient's extreme embodiment, coupled with the nurse's disembodiment, severs relationship (Gadow, 1989).

While torture is rarely discussed as relevant to nursing, analogies can easily be drawn between common acts in torture and common acts in nursing that inflict pain. Nurses participate in a variety of invasive, embarrassing, and painful procedures that cause patients to suffer. What differentiates these acts from torture? In this paper, I will explore this question first by analyzing the basic structure of torture. In addition, I will examine the practice of nurses disembodying in order not to suffer while inflicting pain, and the consequences of such disembodiment to the nurse-patient relationship. Only the nurse's conscious attempts to remain embodied while inflicting pain enables caring relationship and differentiates the act from torture.

ABOUT PAIN AND TORTURE

The experience of feeling severe pain is one of extreme embodiment for the sufferer. No means of transcendence enables the sufferer to escape the immediate sense of the body which is in pain. Pain, however, is difficult for onlookers to recognize, for it is inexpressible. Scarry (1985) describes how pain brings about a state anterior to language, for the sounds of pain are universal but prearticulate. Although no words are able to convey severe pain, screams, moans, grunts, cries, and other sounds are universal and irrespective of articulate language. Yet surprisingly, despite the universality of the sounds of pain, pain easily disappears from the onlooker's recognition due to its inability to be communicated in articulate language. Central to pain's inexpressibility is the profound interiority of pain: all other interior states (to wish for, to love whom, to hate what) bring the interior state into recognition. This has implications for its alleviation, for to be alleviated, pain first must be recognized. Pain easily disappears; a central question of Scarry's work is, "How is it that one person can be in the presence of another person in pain and not know it—not know it to the point where he himself inflicts it, and goes on inflicting it?" (p. 12). The ability to deny pain, to "not know" of another's pain is fundamental to the structure of torture.

Torture is the intentional infliction of pain, and is the one human act which is unambiguously and nearly universally construed as evil (Gadow, 1990). The structure of torture includes the intentional infliction of pain to reach a goal (in political torture, this goal is often loyalty to the regime, seeking of information, etc.). The process of inflicting pain is objectified into a means to an end by the inflictor: the torturer objectifies the subjective attributes of pain as only a means on the road to a certain goal. In order not to suffer with the victim, the torturer disembodies, or dissociates, with his own body while inflicting pain. With the torturer's disembodiment, the ability to deny the victim's pain arises: the victim's body (and the victim) are objectified and the reality of the victim's pain denied. It is this process of disembodiment and the resulting inability to recognize the victim's pain that severs the human relationship and allows the process of torture to continue. The torturer inflicts the pain, objectifies the pain into a means to an end, and then denies the pain through his own disembodiment. Scarry (1985) writes: ". . . and only this final act of self-blinding permits the shift back to the first step, the inflicting of still more pain, for to allow the reality of the other's suffering to enter his own consciousness would immediately compel him to stop the torture" (p. 57). Relationship cannot exist between the torturer and victim, for the extreme embodiment of the victim, coupled with the disembodiment of the torturer, creates a chasm which cannot be bridged (Gadow, 1989, p. 540). This severance of human relationship is central to the torturer's ability to continue to torture despite the victim's verbal and physical expressions of agony (see Table 1).

Table 1
The Basic Structure of Torture

The torturer inflicts pain as a means to a "good" end. This enables the torturer to deny the victim's pain by focusing on the future "good" to be obtained.

The torturer disembodies, or dissociates with his own body in order to avoid suffering with the victim. The victim's body (and victim) are regarded as objects; the subjective attributes of being human are denied the victim.

The process of denial of pain through the disembodiment of the torturer and objectification of the victim enables the torturer to continue to inflict pain in spite of the victim's suffering.

PRACTICES COMMON TO TORTURE AND NURSING

In an article on torture, Laborde (1989) described common forms of torture in third world countries: physical torture includes the infliction of physical pain on another by burns, wounds, sleep deprivation, immobilization, starvation, thirst, and so on. Psychological torture includes psychological pain such as sensory deprivation (isolation, solitary confinement, deprivation of social contact); sensory overload (constant exposure to bright lights or noise), and treating the victim as a nonhuman object. Pharmacological torture includes victims being given drugs which cause painful physiological or psychological effects.

Laborde's listing of common practices of torture seems uncomfortably close to many acts which nurses "routinely" perform. In pursuit of myriad goals, nurses perform invasive and embarrassing procedures which cause patients physical and psychological pain: venipunctures, catherizations, irrigations, dressing changes, feeding tube insertions, wound and burn debridement, repeated vaginal examinations of women in labor, turning and ambulating patients after surgery, and immobilization of limbs for medical procedures or safety. Nurses often must deny tired patients rest, hungry and thirsty patients food and/or water. In modern hospitals, a pervasive theme is the treatment of patients as objects: the patient becomes a body with a disease rather than a subjective human being who is suffering a disease. Patient privacy and modesty often are subjugated in the name of medical convenience, and anxious patients often are made to wait for long periods of time before they receive appropriate medical treatment and nursing care. Laboring women in pain, for one, are sometimes left alone for long periods of time. After birth, their babies are routinely taken from them, even as they nurse, to wait in the nursery for pediatric examinations. When other kinds of patients are kept isolated from others and visitors restricted, sensory deprivation occurs. In intensive care units, where too few attempts are made to reduce constant bright lights or noise, sensory overload is common. Patients who are "difficult," noncompliant, or seem to have more pain than the situation warrants may be ridiculed, ignored, or given placebos. In addition, nurses are the usual administrators of drugs which are known for their distressing effects, such as chemotherapeutic agents for cancer therapy or betaminetics to inhibit preterm labor.

In 1978, Mary Daley described nurses as the "token torturers" (p. 277) of the health care system. Daley discussed how nurses are visible agents of pain, while physicians remain invisible and distanced by merely "ordering" nurses to carry out painful treatments and procedures. While physicians and surgeons usually anesthetize patients when performing painful procedures, the techniques of even local anesthesia are considered outside the domain of nursing. As such, most procedures experienced as painful by patients are done by nurses. As Dind states (1989), "Hurting is part of the job (p. 81)."

But what of the nurse's good intentions? Nurses inflict pain for a variety of reasons, most of which involve some form of eventual "good" (usually improved health or lessened pain in the future) for their patients. However, intent to "do good" does not differentiate nursing practices from torture, for the torturer, too, intends what he perceives as a "good" (gaining of information, loyalty, etc.). Both the torturer's and the nurse's goals of doing "good" may be far removed from the victim or patient's conception of good. The overriding goals of both torturer and nurse deny the sufferer's experience of pain by objectifying it into a means to an end. Relationship is severed, and the inflictor is able to continue to inflict pain despite the sufferer's obvious suffering. (For an eloquent discussion on intentions and nursing relationship, see Gadow, 1986.)

THE PROCESS OF INFLICTING PAIN
IN NURSING

How do nurses cope with the reality of constantly performing acts which cause another human being suffering? Although the infliction of pain is a large part of nursing care, little attention is given to the process in nursing education, practice, or research. In nursing education, painful procedures are considered "skills" or tasks to be mastered, relegated to skills labs and practice on mannequins. Technical competence is all, while little or no encouragement is offered students on ways to remain in relationship with patients while inflicting pain. Many times, the most junior faculty member is placed in charge of skills "labs," and little precedent exists to encourage faculty to help students reflect on the meaning of inflicting pain in nursing. In nursing practice, the methods of natural science, which encourage objectification and distancing, are the basis of medical and much of nursing care. Here, natural science relegates the process of inflicting pain during medical treatments to a "necessary evil," only a means on the road to a certain goal (health, cure, the seeking of information for diagnosis, lessened pain in the future, etc.). Technical competence also is much admired by both nurses and physicians; too much reflection on the consequences and meanings of inflicting pain often is considered only a dangerous route to burnout. "The end is worthy of the means," "somebody has to do it," and "the benefit outweighs the risk" are common rejoinders to parents, patients, or novice nurses who protest the suffering which accompanies much of modern medical and nursing treatments. Novice nurses are encouraged to remain professional (and distanced) by focusing on the future good to be obtained for the patient rather than the morally ambiguous process of hurting another human being. Nurse researchers, while studying and documenting in some detail the processes of nurses relieving pain and the failure of nurses to recognize and treat pain, have done little research on the process of nurses inflicting pain, or on ways for nurses to remain in relationship while hurting another human being.

Because so little attention is given by education, practice, or research on the process of inflicting pain in nursing, nurses are little equipped to remain in relationship with their patients while performing painful procedures. To avoid suffering with their patients, nurses quickly learn to disembody, or separate from their own body while inflicting pain. A distressing consequence occurs as a result of this process: by disembodying to avoid suffering, the patient's experience of pain is denied and nurse–patient relationship severed. By disembodying, nurses are able to remain onlookers (Buber, 1965) and are able to refuse or mask accountability for their actions. Because of this process, disembodied nurses usually fail to recognize or treat the pain and accompanying separation and helplessness patients feel as a consequence of nurses' actions. This severance of relationship by nurses with its concomitant refusal of accountability is the process which converts medically authorized pain into nursing torture. Sally Tisdale (1986) writes:

> I suspect that easing the suffering of others is always inconvenient. To do so, one must stop deflecting the pain, stop the evasion, take the nose up from the ground. The fact remains that much — not a little — of modern medical treatment is painful and damaging in and of itself and that as this pain increases, so does our sense of powerlessness . . . . We are restless and can't name the cause. We wash the faces of peoples hanging by their toes over death and think of . . . something else. (p. 11)

ALTERNATIVES TO NURSING TORTURE: CARING AS EMBODIED RELATIONSHIP

When the nurse–patient relationship is viewed as primary, the basic structure of torture cannot occur. Conceptualizing caring in nursing as relationship without outcome, engagement with no purpose, ensures that relationship remains at the forefront of nurse–patient interactions. When relationship is all, the nurse–patient relationship can be negotiated between nurse and patient depending on the needs of the patient at each encounter. Unlike relationships in natural science, no formula exists for the nursing relationship, for it is the subjectivity of the patient and nurse together which determines the characteristics of the relationship.

Another alternative to torture in nursing is for nurses to consciously re-inhabit their own bodies (Gadow, 1989), especially when performing painful procedures. As Gadow discusses, while a disembodied nurse may be invulnerable to pain, the nurse also is immune to relationship. Embodiment means vulnerability; but it also means the potential exists for human connection. Conveying this vulnerability is one way of expressing the nurse's embodiment to patients in pain. Nurses who find the words to convey their fear, anguish, or bewilderment about the situation open the door to relationship, for only then are the nurse and patient able to mutually search for meanings. No longer does an external framework (such as natural science) console the nurse at the expense of the concrete experience of the patient. Viewing illness as experience to be lived, rather than to be eradicated, encourages nurses to remain in relationship with patients while inflicting pain. This view encourages the search for subjective meaning in the experience of illness and pain. Perhaps most importantly, when relationship is all, conscious embodiment encourages nurses to recognize and reflect on the inhumanity of much of the "caring" that is modern nursing practice. If a nursing procedure is so abhorrent that nurses can only perform it as disembodied beings, protecting themselves from the pain they create by denying relationship, then this procedure is open to challenge.

Other alternatives to disembodiment in nursing arise from nursing's liberation from obsolete ways of knowing and doing that stem from the natural science paradigm that rules medicine and much of nursing. Few schools of nursing include any formal courses on pain (Graffam, 1990), while all teach courses on nursing "skills." Courses on pain which include content on ways nurses manage to remain embodied while inflicting pain would be of assistance to students dismayed at many of the procedures they must perform. Encouraging students to try to find individual meaning in the experience of inflicting pain should be valued; "technical competence" should not be the only criteria instructors place on the performance of skills.

Schools of nursing are just beginning to value ways of knowing outside of traditional science. In this effort, literature, poetry, and story are particularly rich forms of narrative knowing which can enable nurses to vicariously experience and reflect on the process of inflicting and experiencing pain. Through narrative, nurses may be better able to devise creative ways to remain in relationship with patients no matter what the circumstance. Liberated from a focus on natural science, nurses can begin to realize that the caring relationship resides in the challenge of continual questioning of the beliefs and methods of nursing. In this way, responsibility for nursing actions which results in another's suffering is affirmed rather than denied; embodied nurses are compelled to recognize and confront the moral ambiguities inherent in nursing practice. Rather than one truth based in natural science, everything has a truth based in the contradictions of embodied existence.

When relationship is primary, the process of nurses inflicting pain returns to what it is, a morally ambiguous act, often an unavoidable— but never routine—part of nursing practice. By attempting to remain in relationship while inflicting pain, the basic structure of torture cannot occur in nursing. By remaining true to that which we know as nurses, we can begin to reclaim that what we know as ours: nursing as a caring relationship. If embodied relationship were considered primary in nursing, perhaps nurses would no longer be accused of being the token torturers of the health care system.

REFERENCES

Buber, M. (1965). *Between man and man.* New York: Macmillan.

Daley, M. (1978). *Gyn/Ecology: The metaethics of radical feminism.* Boston: Beacon Press.

Dind, C. (1989). Teaching nurses about torture. *International Nursing Review, 36*(3), 81–82.

Gadow, S. (1986). Robots, despots, and cronys. *Humanities and the health professions, 8,* (17–27).

Gadow, S. (1989). Clinical subjectivity: Advocacy with silent patients. *Nursing Clinics of North America, 24*(12), 535–541.

Gadow, S. (1990). Remembered in the body: Pain and moral uncertainty. In C. Kliever (Ed.), *Essays in medical ethics and human meaning* (pp. 151–167). Dallas, TX: S. Methodist & University Press.

Graffam, S. (1990). Pain content in the curriculum: A survey. *Nurse Educator, 14*(1), 20–23.

Laborde, J. (1989). Torture: A nursing concern. *Image, 21* (1), 31–33.

Newman, M., Sime, M., & Corcoran-Perry. (1991). The focus of the discipline of nursing. *Advances in Nursing Science, 14*(1), 1–6.

Scarry, E. (1985). *The body in pain: The making and unmaking of the world.* New York: Oxford Press.

Tisdale, S. (1986). *The sorcerer's apprentice: Medical miracles and other disasters.* New York: Henry Holt and Co.

Veazeu, T. & Schroeder, C. (1991). Caring approaches: A critical examination of origin, balance of power, embodiment, time and space, and intended outcome. In P. Chinn (Ed.), *Anthology on caring (pp. 1–16).* New York: National League of Nursing.

15

A Caring Presence: Confederate Nursing Practice

Sylvia Rinker

K ate Cumming, Confederate nurse between 1862 and 1865, had her own ideas about the "woman's sphere" that was popularly discussed in her nineteenth-century Southern society: "In war, the men are to fight and the women's *true* sphere is to nurse the wounded and sick" (1975, p. 123). The women who dared step outside their "acceptable sphere" (i.e., the home) demonstrated a compassionate caring that was to help shape a new world, not only for the victims of war, but also for women and for nursing. The purpose of this historical study of written documents left by women who served as nurses in the Confederacy is to uncover how their experiences as nineteenth-century women caring for soldiers impacted early nursing practice. Their compassionate response to the agonizing conditions of war will be examined; their creative and competent reinterpretation of their society's expectations of "true womanhood" in order to care for sick and wounded men will be delineated; and finally, examples of how their nursing practice demonstrates essential attributes of caring as defined by Roach (1987) will be given.

A woman from Georgia who was present during the Civil War cried out: "It's wrong—all war is wrong! It is not only the fighting and killing—it's what it does to the souls. . ." (Hodnett, 1917, p. 67). Southern women responded to the needs of the "souls" afflicted by war in ways that were to dispel forever the position designated them by their nineteenth-century society as "weak women." The untrained women who served as nurses in the Confederacy possessed, concomitant with their "weak woman" status, certain "womanly virtues," which they used in powerful ways in the midst of the chaos of war by being there to provide a caring presence for its victims. Their caring for soldiers, expressed in their willingness to be fully present, produced powerful results, very much in contrast with what could have been expected from their own self-description as "weak women." Patricia Benner (1984) has introduced the idea that there is power in the caring of nurses for their patients. Confederate nurses' personal experiences, reported in their own words through diaries and letters, give evidence of this power, emerging from their caring for soldiers. The "weak women" who left a record of their lives during the war were mostly white, middle and upper-class women. Thus, it is their experience that is explored in this paper, with the full recognition that poor white women and black women (Carnegie, 1984) also have both a story and an impact on the world as we live it today.

CONDITIONS OF WAR

Mary Chesnut's experience with war was graphically expressed in 1866: "There are nights here with the moonlight cold and ghastly when I could tear my hair and cry aloud for all that is past and gone" (1984, p. xxii). Her anguished cry was for the disintegration of her cherished southern world, courtesy of the Civil War. Her anguish was well-founded; the transition of the country from peace to the tumult and waste of war, appalling and swift, profoundly changed the world of the southern woman. A white population of about five-and-a-half million Southerners provided armed forces of about one-million men (Wiley, 1975, p. 154). That meant that families who sent no one to war were rare, and that those who provided several were not uncommon. Susan Blackford stated simply: "Lincoln's call for troops changed the whole course of our ordinary lives" (1947, p. 5).

Medical Knowledge and Practice

At the time of the Civil War, medical knowledge and practice were primitive and unscientific (Parsons, 1983). In fact, an entire medical education could be had in less than a year.

> *With little or no training and experience in military medicine or surgery . . . the medical staff was faced with the grave responsibility of caring for more than three million cases of disease and wounds in an invaded and blockaded country. (Cunningham, 1958, p. 11)*

Only one-third of the 258,000 deaths in the Confederate military forces were properly attributable to the results of battle; it was disease that was the chief killer—taking the lives of approximately 164,000 Southern soldiers (Robertson, 1988, p. 147). One soldier wrote: "Those Big Battles is not as bad as the fevers" (Brooks, 1966, p. 6).

The treatment of wounds was not particularly successful either. The ignorance of antisepsis is clear in this description by Civil War surgeon, William Keen: "We operated in our old blood-stained and often pus-stained coats, the veterans of a hundred fights. We used undisinfected instruments from undisinfected plush cases. We probed chest or abdominal wounds with our fingers, prescribed morphine, and tried to stop external bleeding" (Stevenson, 1941, p. 918). Not surprisingly, the frequent amputations performed during the Civil War posed a terminal threat to most of the soldiers who suffered them. Mrs. Pember (1987) went so far as to state that the only cases under her observation who survived amputations ". . . were Irishmen, and it was really so difficult to kill an Irishman," she claimed, "that there was little cause for boasting on the part of the surgeon" (p. 77).

Unexpected Length and Devastation

Not only did the length of the war catch the nation by surprise; neither government was prepared for the onslaught of sick and wounded soldiers the war would produce (Rogge, 1985, p. 32). After the battles, the nearby villages or towns were crowded with wounded and dying men who were placed in makeshift hospitals that were established in barns, hotels, churches, and warehouses. Susan Blackford (1947) describes the scene on May 12, 1864, in Lynchburg, Virginia:

> I heard Toliaferro's warehouse was full of soldiers in a deplorable condition. I went down there with a bucket of rice milk, a basin, towel, soap, etc. to see what I could do. I found the house filled with wounded men and not one thing provided for them. They are lying about the floor on a little straw. I washed and dressed the wounds of about fifty and poured water over the wounds of many more . . . If it had not been for the ladies many of the men would have starved to death. (p. 259)

These scenes multiplied as the war continued, forcing Southern women to overcome their "rightful delicacy" that dying men might be comforted. And the pain was not only physical. Fiercely patriotic statements such as that of Mary Chesnut—"We separated North from South because of incompatibility of temper. We are divorced because we have hated each other so" (1961, p. 108)—could not erase the underlying feeling so well expressed by Mrs. Robert E. Lee: ". . . both parties are wrong in this fratricidal war. I see no *right* in the matter" (1988, p. 23). Such were the conditions under which the Southern woman found herself compelled to nurse at the outset of the war. She used her womanly virtues very effectively, in the fulfillment of her new responsibilities.

TRUE WOMANHOOD OF NINETEENTH-CENTURY WOMEN

Several historians (Fox-Genovese, 1988; Faust, 1990; Lebsock, 1984) have provided insight into the conflicts faced by nineteenth-

century American women, subject to the ideology of the time concerning "true womanhood." This ideology defined women as innately
different from men—intellectually inferior, more submissive and re-
tiring, purer, more pious and morally sensitive, and "by nature"
domestic and maternal (Welter, 1966). Given these unalterable differences, woman was to inhabit and confine herself to her own separate
and distinct "sphere," that of the home. Kerber (1988) has noted,
however, that this ideology could be both prescriptive *and* instrumental. While it was experienced as constricting, it also was found to
be a comfortable link for Southern women, between their old familiar
world and the one torn apart by war. Regardless of how the ideology
of true womanhood was interpreted, the Civil War, in its relentless
power and fury, required a whole new set of behaviors of Southern
women. Their response to this upheaval, their presence in caring for
the victims of war, proved to be powerful in unexpected ways, for the
women, for their patients, and for nursing itself.

Nursing in the Nineteenth Century

It is estimated that 1,000 Southern women were engaged in nursing and hospital administration during the Civil War (Maher, 1989).
The step taken to enter nursing in the nineteenth century was
indeed a steep, hazardous step, for the nineteenth-century hospital
was "hospitable" neither to women nor to patients! Only those who
had no family to care for them entered the hospitals (Rogge, 1985).
The hapless patient had to rely on aged inmates, derelicts, or down-
and-outs who could not find a job doing anything else. Few people
worth their salt entered the "profession," and certainly *no lady!* For
the first year and a half of the War, Southern women worked in the
hospitals as volunteers. On September 27, 1862, Congress granted
them official status (U.S. War Department, *Official Records of the
War of the Rebellion*, 1880–1901, p. 221).

With the men away at war, "woman's sphere" suddenly became
very elastic (Scott, 1970) and thus her womanly virtues required a new
interpretation and application as she began to look beyond the constricting walls of her "woman's sphere." The women who responded
to the call to "be there" for sick and wounded soldiers transcended

their nineteenth-century societal expectations in courageous, caring practices that not only humanized the devastation of war for its victims, but also elevated the status of women and nursing.

Obstacles.   These newly sanctioned hospital workers faced a variety of obstacles as they began their work. One of the greatest obstacles was the fact that most bedside nursing was done by enlisted men, convalescent from illness or wounds. As convalescents, they were themselves unable to do heavy work, and as rapidly as they became stronger they were ordered back to the front, so that attendants were constantly changing, always untrained, and requiring constant supervision (Cunningham, 1958). Kate Cumming (1975) noted early in the war a need for education for nursing. She was frustrated with the continual turnover of the male nurses at her hospital:

> *I cannot see how it is possible for them to take proper care of the men, as nursing is a thing that has to be learned, and we should select our best men for it—the best, not physically, but morally—as I am certain that none but good, conscientious persons will ever do justice to the patients. (p. 7)*

A general prejudice against women was another obstacle the Confederate women who responded to the call to care for the sick and wounded had to face. One of Pheobe Pember's (1987) first experiences upon her arrival at Chimborazo Hospital was hearing "the little contract surgeon" inform one of his friends, "in a tone of ill-concealed disgust that 'one of them' (women) had come" (p. 17). The ire and indignity this prejudice against women aroused is expressed by Kate Cumming (1975): "Not respectable! . . . it is useless to say the surgeons will not allow us; we have our rights, and if asserted properly, will get them. This is our right (to care for soldiers) and ours alone!" (p. 55). Rogge (1985) has aptly explained it: Surgeons might oppose them, and refined sensibilities might be offended, but one fact was undeniable: the women were more capable, by virtue of their domestic training, to nurse the war's casualties than were convalescent soldiers or detail attendants (p. 66).

Nuns.   The only class of women in the South who possessed formal training in nursing were the Roman Catholic Sisterhoods (Cunningham, 1958). Martin (1961) notes that:

Responding to requests from the Surgeons General of both Union and Confederacy, they went wherever suffering humanity could be found and cared impartially for all. Their ability to carry out instructions, to administer medicines and prepare meals on schedule, and to maintain cleanliness, order, and quiet in the wards was appreciated by the overworked Army surgeons on both sides. (p. 550)

Six hundred and seventeen Sisters from 21 different communities representing 12 separate orders nursed both Union and Confederate soldiers (Maher, 1989).

They gave drink to parched lips, administered medicines, bound up flowing wounds, and soothed the last moments of the dying . . . When there were not enough bandages, the Sisters unhesitatingly tore strips from their own garments. To the wounded, it was holy fabric from angels in hell. (Robinson, 1946, p. 177)

Being There: Caring via Womanly Attributes

As their gentile Southern society crumbled around them, the female nurses of the Confederacy found it necessary to reinterpret their womanly attributes. They did so most effectively, through the caring presence they provided the victims of war.

Domesticity. Though the other virtues were "expected," the September 1862 Law required that matrons superintend the entire domestic economy of the hospital. Pember (1987) noted: "I, upon reading the bill, could only understand that the office (of matron) was one that dovetailed the duties of housekeeper and cook, nothing more" (p. 20). The preparation of food for the sick and wounded was a first duty performed by both Cumming and Pember upon their arrivals at their respective hospitals.

Kate Cumming: "The first thing I did was to aid in giving the men their supper, consisting of bread, biscuit, butter, and tea and coffee, without milk." (p. 6)

Phoebe Pember: " . . . in the meantime, chicken soup was boiling . . . Nature may not have intended me for a Florence Nightingale, but a kitchen proved my worth." (p. 20)

Phoebe Pember concocted a mint julep for a supposedly dying man, who decided, based on that drink, that as long as 1st proof brandy and mint lasted in the Confederacy, this world was good enough for him—he *lived!* (p. 77). However, the scarcity of "victuals" was a constant concern for the matrons. Kate Cumming wrote: "One of our greatest trials is want of proper diet for sick men" (p. 57). The frustration and compassion Phoebe Pember felt at this deprivation is clearly expressed as she thoughtfully commented: "Battles fought by starving the sick and wounded . . . by crushing in day by day all the necessities of human nature, make victories hardly worth the name" (p. 61).

Another important component of the domesticity virtue was that of cleanliness. Cumming (1975) noted: "There could be great improvement in the laundry department. The men's dirty clothes are taken off when they come in, put in their haversacks, and put back on—bloody and filthy as they were—when they leave the hospital" (p. 85). Confederate female nurses used their domesticity virtue not only to do the laundry, but also to cleanse grotesque, life-threatening wounds. The crowded conditions made cleanliness very difficult. Kate Cumming describes one scene:

The men are lying all over the house . . . just as they were brought in from the battlefield . . . . The foul air from this mass of human beings at first made me sick. When we give the men anything we have to kneel in blood and water . . . (p. 6)

The domesticity virtue also included a woman's responsibility to cheer and comfort the soldiers' minds—and this they did amidst the agony of war. The Southern matrons wrote letters for their patients, sent locks of hair to their families, and at times even buried the bodies in special places. They made no distinction, when treating wounded men, whether they were of their own side or the enemy's. Mrs. Newsom found a severely wounded soldier who said to her: "You wouldn't be so kind if you knew . . . I am on the enemy's side." "But," said she, "you are fallen and I make no distinction" (Richard, 1914, p. 55).

Submission.   The womanly virtue of submission during the war was expressed as a submission to the "duty" of woman to care for the sick; accepting this responsibility often required less than submissive behaviors, however. There was a general acceptance of the surgeon's superiority, but in many instances of his absence or his incompetence, the female nurses acted in a decidedly unsubmissive manner. Miss Emily Mason, of Lexington, Virginia, relates the story of her "dead men":

> *In another ward lay upon the floor two young men just taken from an ambulance dead, as was supposed. Their heads were enveloped in bloody bandages and the little clothing they had was glued to their bodies with mud and gravel. Hastily examining them, the surgeon ordered them to the "Dead House." I prayed they might be left until morning . . . as neither of them had the rigidity of death in their limbs. The surgeon pointed to the wounds below the ear, the jaws shattered, and one or both eyes put out, and reminded me that even could they be brought back to life it would be an existence worse than death.*
>
> *"Life is sweet," I replied, "even to the blind and the deaf and dumb, and these men may be the darlings of some fond hearts who will love them more in their helplessness than in their sunniest hours."*

And so I kept my "dead men" (1885, p. 157). Her "unsubmissiveness" was rewarded, and though one of the men "never recovered his mind, which had been shattered with his body," the other one recovered sufficiently to "marry and live happily ever after."

The matrons in the hospitals *did* submissively follow the doctor's orders. Kate Cumming (1975) declared: "The surgeons alone are responsible for the sick under their control and have the right to direct what should be done for them" (p. 123).

Purity.   Before the war, entering a hospital filled with strange men would have constituted an automatic death-knell to the Southern woman's precious purity. Kate Cumming confessed her fears in 1862: "For awhile I wavered about the propriety of going into the hospital" (p. 55). She became much more emphatic a year later declaring ". . . a lady's respectability must be at a low ebb when it can be endangered by going into a hospital!" (p. 123). She continued, ". . . in truth, none but the 'refined and modest' have any business in the hospitals!" Pember (1987) sums it up:

> In the midst of suffering and death, praying by the bedside of the lonely and heart-stricken; closing the eyes of boys hardly old enough to realize a man's sorrows, much less suffer by man's fierce hate, a woman must soar beyond the conventional modesty considered correct under different circumstances. (p. 105)

Piety.   Permeating all the womanly virtues of the Southern woman, bearing her up under her excruciating losses, and providing her a rock in her destroyed world, was her unwavering belief in her God. Often the most patriotic statements are directly linked to God: "I will play my part with courage, seeing I have been deemed worthy, by the God who made me, to suffer in this sublime struggle for liberty" (Pryor, 1988, p. 60). Kate Cumming (1975) allowed, however, that the war had made of her ". . . certainly not the better Christian, for I love the enemies less than ever!" (p. 125). As a nurse, she often prayed with her patients, and attended services in the hospital wards (p. 163). Phoebe Pember (1987) realized, when she had reached her limitations in caring for a man whose wound was "right through the body," that there was only one more thing she could do: "What comfort could I give? Only silently open the Bible and read to him without comment the everliving promises of his Maker" (p. 39).

Weak Woman's Power.   The reinterpretation of their womanly virtues to allow Confederate women to care for soldiers had surprising results. Although untrained in nursing, Confederate nurses entered into their nursing caring responsibilities with an expressed willingness "to do all that was in weak woman's power." At the outset of the war, one South Carolina woman said: ". . . we felt forlorn and forsaken, but at the same time the true 'rebel' spirit burned in our hearts and we were ready to do and suffer all that was in weak woman's power" (E.L.L., 1885, p. 251). That power was effective, as evidenced by Sally Tompkins' success at her Robertson Hospital in Richmond. It had the lowest death rate of all the other hospitals in the city:

> The Robertson Hospital was the only private hospital allowed to
> continue its existence after the act of the Confederate Congress
> absorbed all hospitals into the military organization. On July 30,
> 1861, ten days after the first battle of Manassas, Miss Sally L.
> Tompkins opened this hospital, equipping and operating it entirely
> at her own expense. When she learned of the orders which were
> about to close her institution, she appeared before President Jeffer-
> son Davis, displayed the records showing the number of cases
> treated, the low incidence of death, and the high percentage of men
> returned to duty. The president met her appeal by one of the most
> remarkable military orders in history. He created Miss Tompkins a
> captain in the Confederate Army and thus authorized the continu-
> ance of her organization. Records show 1,334 patients were cared
> for at this hospital from August 1, 1861 to April 2, 1865. (Blanton,
> 1933, p. 303)

A real tribute to the impact of women on the care of the sick and
wounded in the hospitals was given by Dr. Welch, Confederate
surgeon, who wrote his wife on August 10, 1863: "Last year when a
soldier was sent to a hospital he was expected to die, but all who
come from the hospitals in Richmond now are highly pleased with
the treatment they received" (Welch, 1954, p. 74).

CARING BY CONFEDERATE NURSES

Confederate nurses came untrained to the formidable task before them. They had not the benefit of education, theoretical
frameworks, or research findings on caring to guide their practice.
Before nursing was defined, Confederate nurses practiced it, offering themselves and all that was in "weak woman's power." The
evidence is that the female nurses of the Confederacy reinter-
preted their womanly duties to allow them to enter fully into
the privilege of "being with" and "caring for" soldiers. They clearly
demonstrated the attributes of caring that Roach (1987) has
identified: compassion, competence, confidence, conscience, and
commitment.

Compassion

Compassion is defined by Roach (1987) as ". . . a way of living born out of an awareness of one's relationship to all living creatures; engendering a response of participation in the experience of another; a sensitivity to the pain and brokenness of the other; a quality of presence which allows one to share with and make room for the other" (p. 58). Compassion moved Confederate women, such as Pheobe Pember, to enter into the places of pain, to share the brokenness, fear, confusion, and anguish. Pember describes the scene at her Chimborazo Hospital in Richmond, in the Spring of 1864:

> *Can any pen or pencil do justice to those squalid pictures of famine and desolation? Those gaunt, lank skeletons with the dried yellow flesh clinging to bones enlarged by dampness and exposure? With beating heart, throbbing head, and icy hands I went among this army whom it was almost impossible to recognize as human beings; powerless to speak, chocking with unavailing pity, but still striving to aid and comfort.* (p. 70)

Impelled by their compassion, Confederate women entered wholeheartedly into a world previously unknown to them, but one that would never again be outside their "acceptable sphere."

Competence

The competence, or ". . . having the knowledge, judgment, skills, energy, experience, and motivation required to respond adequately to one's professional responsibilities" was acquired by Confederate nurses quickly and on the job (Roach, p. 61). Kate Cumming (1975) expressed her trepidation as a brand new matron: "As I had never been where there was a large army, and had never seen a wounded man . . . I could not help feeling a little nervous at the prospect of now seeing both" (p. 5). Her nervousness was well-founded:

I do not think that words are in our vocabulary expressive enough
to present to the mind the realities of that sad scene. Certainly,
none of the glories of war were presented here. But I must not say
that; for if uncomplaining endurance is glory, we had plenty of it. If
it is that which makes the hero, here they were by the scores. Gray-
haired men—men in the pride of manhood—beardless boys—
Federals and all, mutilated in every imaginable way, lying on the
floor, just as they were taken from the battlefield; so close together
it was almost impossible to walk without stepping on them. I could
not command my feelings enough to speak, but thoughts crowded
upon me. (p. 5)

Her response to the scene: "There was work to do; so I went at it to
do what I could." Phoebe Pember said of her first experience in
wound care: "I had been spectator often enough to be skillful"
(p. 38), and that describes the extent of her training for this duty.
The work of Confederate nurses was effective! One measure of their
success is that the death rate in the hospitals managed by women
was 5 percent, whereas, in those managed by men, it was 10 percent.
(Rable, 1989, p. 128).

Competence also required creative approaches to all *sorts* of vex-
ing problems. Emily Mason (1885) describes her use of General
Lee's socks:

Mrs. Lee had given me several pairs of the beloved general's old
socks, so thoroughly darned it was clear they had been well-worn
by our hero. We kept those to apply to those laggard old soldiers
who were suspected of preferring the "luxury" of hospital life to the
activity of the field. Even the threat of General Lee's socks was
sufficient to cure some of the most obstinate chronic cases! (p. 150)

Confidence

The care given sick and wounded soldiers by another group of
women, the religious nuns, demonstrates their ability to inspire
confidence, to foster trusting relationships in their patients (Roach,

1987, p. 63), despite the initial suspicion their strange appearance aroused:

> One Virginia soldier not only refused to take his medicine from the sisters, but struck at them as they passed. When it finally dawned on him that his behavior did not have the slightest effect on their attitude toward him, his curiosity overcame his resentment, and he asked: "What are you?" "I am a Sister of Charity." "Where is your husband?" "I have none, and I am glad I have not." Infuriated at this answer, he demanded: "Why are you glad?" His nurse replied: "Because if I had I would not be here waiting on you." Her enemy turned his face away, humbled, subdued, and utterly vanquished. Upon his recovery, it was noticed he was an ardent champion of the Sisters of Charity. (Robinson, p. 177)

Conscience

Conscience, according to Roach (1987), is a state of moral awareness; a compass directing one's behavior according to the moral fitness of things (p. 64). Kate Cumming (1975) saw the relief of suffering to be ". . . as it has been in all ages, the special duty of woman" (p. 56). Southern women not only responded individually to the needs of their culture in war; they also organized. Simkins and Patton (1936) wrote:

> The same stimulus that prompted the Confederate women to the painful duty of yielding friends and kinsmen to the army also impelled them to assume the burden of providing many of the material comforts and necessities that were indispensable to the equipment and efficiency of the Confederate forces. No armed conflict in the previous history of the race had ever witnessed the organization of civilian relief on so vast a scale as was experienced during the War for Southern Independence. The work of the United States Sanitary Commission, the United States Christian Commission, and other agencies in the North is well known;

*and although not organized to the same extent, the burdens
borne by the non-combatant population in the South were even
greater than in the free states. It is a tribute to feminine sagacity
that the women of the Confederacy understood the significance
and the necessity of these labors. (1936, p. 18)*

Mrs. Sallie Gordon-Law (1894) reports on the efforts of one group
of Confederate women whose conscience directed their behaviors:

*I heard that thousands of soldiers at Dalton, Georgia, were
having to sit up all night round a log fire, for want of blankets. I
was so greatly troubled, that I went directly to a Ladies' Aid
Society. I told what I had heard of the suffering—and boxes of
good things—chicken, ham, sausage, butter, pickles, bread, and
cake were packed, and I carried them to the boys, along with
blankets. (p. 107)*

Commitment

Commitment is defined as a deliberate choice to act in accordance
with the affective response characterized by the convergence between one's desires and one's obligations (Roach, p. 66). The commitment of Confederate women to relieve war's suffering is evident
in the deliberate choices they made to act in accordance with their
new obligations. The dilemma of the Southern woman who responded to her call to duty to relieve the suffering of the sick is
captured by Cumming as she wrote on June 18, 1862: "Men nowa-
days seem to think we women have no right to leave our homes."
But leave their homes they did.

Mrs. Forsberg, of the Ladies' Relief Hospital in Lynchburg, Virginia, recalls an incident which shows the Confederate nurses' willing commitment to her new duties:

*When the trains began arriving with their terrible loads of suf-
fering ones from the battle of the Wilderness, 120 of them were
delivered at the Ladies' Hospital and I was there to help receive*

them. It was my privilege (I thought it so then; I think so still), to
kneel by each stretcher, as it was brought in and placed on the
floor. Raising the occupant's head to my shoulder, I gave him
a tin cup full of iced buttermilk before any questions were asked
as to his name, company, or regiment. (Lynchburg News, 28
Nov. 1920)

CONCLUSION

Confederate women certainly were not immune to the grievous
losses which result from war. The fierce patriotism expressed by
Southern women at the outset of the war was slowly eroded by the
constant deprivation of the lives they were forced to live (Wiley,
1975). The poverty and volatile race relations which characterized
the Reconstruction years nearly suffocated the new opportunities
which had been barely glimpsed by the women of the South (Lebsock, 1984). A good many women, however, submerged the grief of
their days by investing the full force of their "womanly attributes" in
the care of sick and wounded soldiers.

Caring, for the female nurses of the Confederacy, was a genuine,
human response to the desperate suffering which surrounded
them. The energy that is released through caring is evident in Kate
Cumming's (1975): "I have felt I would not exchange places with
anyone" (p. 80), and in Susan Blackford's (1947) "I have never
worked so hard in all my life . . . (caring for wounded), but I
would rather do this than anything else in the world" (p. 259). The
performance of Confederate nurses lends compelling support to
the premise advanced by Roach (1987), Watson (1988), Leininger
(1980), Benner (1984), and others that caring is indeed a human
mode of being and a powerful force for nursing. Through their
presence in Confederate hospitals, women came to be respected
both for their practical genius in organization and for their humane
ministrations (Sheahan, 1980, p. 99). In Confederate hospitals, it
was discovered that good nursing was as important as proper medical attention (Cunningham, 1958, p. 210). The Confederate nurses'
courageous commitment to caring for soldiers ". . . broke down

prejudices, opened doors to women, and set on foot the procession of events that led to the emergence of a new profession for women" (Guyot, 1962, p. 314). The Confederate nurses who dared to "be there," in the face of society's disdain and in the midst of the agony of war nursing soldiers, were caring in the fullest sense of the word. The powerful force of caring emerges from the experience of those who demonstrated their caring best by "being there," declaring: "I would not exchange places with anyone."

REFERENCES

Benner, P. (1984). *From novice to expert.* Menlo Park, CA: Addison Wesley.

Blackford, S. (1947). *Letters from Lee's army.* New York: Barnes & Co.

Blanton, W. (1933). *Medicine in Virginia in the nineteenth century.* Richmond: Garrett & Massie.

Brooks, S. (1966). *Civil war medicine.* Springfield: Thomas.

Carnegie, E. (1984). Black nurses at the front. *American Journal of Nursing, 84,* 1250–1252.

Chesnut, M. (1961). *A diary from Dixie.* Gloucester: Peter Smith.

Chesnut, M. (1866). In C. Van Woodward & E. Muhlenfeld, (Eds.), *The private Mary Chesnut.* (1984). New York: Oxford University.

Cumming, K. (1975). *The journal of Kate Cumming: A confederate nurse 1862–1865.* R. Harwell (Ed.). Savannah: The Beehive Press.

Cunningham, H. (1958). *Doctors in gray.* Baton Rouge: Louisiana State University Press.

Faust, D. (1990). Altars of sacrifice: Confederate women and the narratives of war. *The Journal of American History, 76,* 1200–1228.

Forsberg, A. (1920, 28 November). Lynchburg hospitals of the past. *Lynchburg News.*

Fox-Genovese, E. (1988). *Within the plantation household.* Chapel Hill: University of North Carolina.

Gordon-Law, (April 1894). Reminiscences—Mother of the Confederacy. *Confederate Veteran,* 105–108.

Guyot, H. (1962). The nurse in civil war literature. *Nursing Outlook, 10,* 311–314.

Hodnett, M. (1917). Hodnett Family Papers, Atlanta Historical Society. In C. Kunkle (1989, Summer). It is what it does to the souls. *Atlanta History,* 57–70.

Kerber, L. (1988). Separate spheres, female worlds, woman's place: The rhetoric of women's history. *The Journal of American History, 75,* 9–39.

L., E.L. (1885). Troublous times. In *Our women in the war.* Charleston: The News and Courier Books Presses.

Lebsock, S. (1984). *The free women of Petersburg.* New York: W. W. Norton & Co.

Lee, M. (1988). The prospects before us are sad. In K. Jones (Ed.), *Heroines of Dixie: Spring of high hopes.* Mockingbird Books, 23.

Leininger, M. (1980). Caring: A central focus of nursing and health care services. *Nursing and Health Care, 1,* 135–143, 176.

Maher, M. (1989). *To bind up the wounds.* New York: Greenwood Press.

Martin, R. (1961). They served the sick in North and South. *Military Medicine, 126,* 547–550.

Mason, E. (1885). Hospital scenes. In *Our women in the war.* Charleston: The News and Courier Books Presses.

Parsons, M. (1983). Mothers and matrons. *Nursing Outlook, 31,* 274–278.

Pember, P. (1987). *A southern woman's story.* Mockingbird Books.

Pryor, S. (1988). Christmas in Petersburg. In K. Jones (Ed.), *Heroines of Dixie: Winter of desperation.* Mockingbird Books.

Rable, G. (1989). *Civil wars: Women and the crisis of southern nationalism.* Urbana, IL: University of Illinois Press.

Richard, J. Fraise. (1914). *The Florence Nightingale of the southern army: Experiences of Mrs. Ella K. Newsom, confederate nurse.* New York: Broadway Publishing.

Roach, M. (1987). *The human act of caring.* Toronto: Canadian Hospital Association.

Robertson, J. (1988). *Soldiers blue and gray.* Columbia: University of South Carolina Press.

Robinson, V. (1946). *White caps.* Philadelphia: J.B. Lippincott.

Rogge, M. (1985). *Development of a taxonomy of nursing interventions.* Doctoral dissertation. Austin, TX: The University of Texas at Austin.

Scott, A. (1970). *The southern lady: From pedestal to politics.* Chicago: University of Chicago Press.

Sheahan, D. (1980). *The social origins of American nursing and its movement into the university.* Doctoral dissertation. New York University.

Simkins, F., & Patton, J. (1936). *The women of the confederacy.* Richmond, VA: Garrett & Massie.

Stevenson, I. (1941). Nursing in the civil war. *Ciba Symposia, 3,* 908–918.

U.S. War Department. (1880–1901). *The war of the rebellion: A compilation of the official records of the union and confederate armies.* Washington DC: U.S. Government Printing Office. Series II, Vol. VII, 221.

Watson, J. (1988). *Human science and human care: A theory of nursing.* New York: National League for Nursing.

Welch, S. (1954). *A confederate surgeon's letters to his wife.* Marietta: Continental Book Company.

Welter, B. (1966). The cult of true womanhood: 1820–1860. *American Quarterly, 18,* 151–174.

Wiley, B. (1975). *Confederate women.* Westport, CT: Greenwood Press.

16

The Historical Conflict between Caring and Professionalization: A Dilemma for Nursing

Kathryn Gardner

Although in the last few decades nurses have made considerable progress toward professionalization, nursing remains classified as an emerging, or minor, profession. A major factor which has influenced nursing progress toward professionalization is its association with caring. In this paper, I will examine how the caring dimension in nursing has conflicted with the professionalization process. To accomplish this, I will summarize the historical status of caring in nursing and critique caring as a characteristic of the nursing profession.

DEFINITION OF CARING

For this review, *caring* includes those processes and activities in nursing directed at meeting patient needs through individualized services. Caring is thus culture specific (Leininger, 1984), focused on interpersonal relationships (Watson, 1985), and calls for a personal commitment which includes individual attention, concern, and attachment (Gaut, 1983). Gaut listed three conditions necessary for caring:

1. Awareness and knowledge of the care receivers' need for care.
2. An intention of the caregiver to act and actions based on knowledge.
3. A positive change in the recipient of care as a result of caring solely on the basis of the welfare of others.

AN EVOLUTION OF CARING IN NURSING

From primitive society until the present time, caring has been an important aspect in nursing. Throughout centuries the practice of nursing has focused on caring for, caring about, and caring with persons, as well as assisting in the curing of persons.

According to Dolan (1985), the goals of nursing in the first centuries were to keep people healthy and to provide comfort, care, and reassurance. Nursing was not extended to all persons, but only to those who demonstrated an ability to care for others. In ancient cultures, nurses became divided about caring. Some cultures, such as the Babylonians, took away the independent and caring practice of nursing, treated nurses as slaves, made them dependent on the physician, and allowed them to perform only custodial care. In contrast, other cultures such as the ancient Hebrew continued to focus on the caring aspect of nursing.

Christianity, in highlighting love and charity, made caring the central aspect of nursing. Early Christian nurses enjoyed a high social status and were independent practitioners (Dolan, 1985). Christianity viewed nursing as relieving suffering and providing care. These nurses, many of whom were men, were concerned with the spiritual, physical, and mental health of their patients and families. However, by the seventeenth century in most western cultures, the caring aspects of nursing diminished. Hospitals deteriorated and nursing, except within religious orders, was primarily done by mothers.

In the nineteenth century, Nightingale (1964) emphasized that the purpose of nursing was to restore and promote health and prevent disease. She described nursing as an act of charity, which had an independent knowledge base concerned with the health, comfort, and welfare of patients. Nightingale embryologically promoted the science of nursing and combined this science with the maternal caring attributes of women.

According to Palmer (1983), Nightingale believed that nurses possessed three basic motives: a natural motive or love for nursing the sick, a professional or intellectual motive, and a spiritual motive. Because of the natural and spiritual motive, Nightingale emphasized the duty to care (Reverby, 1990), and rejected economics as a primary concern to advance nursing. She did not advocate that nursing should have a professional organization. However, Nightingale did state that nurses should be paid according to the market price of their labor, receive merit increases, and be given a month's vacation (Palmer, 1983).

Since the time of Nightingale's influence, these two dimensions, science and humanistic caring, while an integral part of nursing, have often been in conflict with each other—a conflict frequently expressed in the care/cure dichotomy. Economic factors in nursing also have been a critical determinant in the development of caring.

According to Lynaugh and Fagin (1988), in the United States the caring aspect of nursing has been undervalued. From the middle of the nineteenth century until the middle of the twentieth century, emphasis was generally placed on the technical and scientific aspects of nursing which resulted in an emphasis on curing functions within structured hospital settings.

Three factors accounted for the shift from a caring to a curing focus. First, nursing was usually under the control and supervision of physicians whose primary intent was to cure. Second, nurses were educated in hospitals with curricula geared toward the medical model. Third, while nursing was historically committed to caring, nurses practiced in institutions which valued curing rather than caring. These pressures resulted in a certain dilemma and a tension in nursing, and especially, as practiced in the hospital. As a result, many nurses became more comfortable and attracted to practicing nursing in homes rather than in the hospital.

However, with urbanization and the increase in medical technology, hospitals became the largest employer of nurses. By the mid-1930s, the autonomy of nursing in private practice was overcome by institutional nursing (Aydelotte, 1983). With the combination of increased medical technology and nurses anchored (or rooted) in the hospital setting, curing rather than caring remained the dominant theme. Nurses who were attracted to emphasizing caring quietly implemented these practice activities, turned to other non-traditional settings to practice nursing, or left the profession entirely.

As nursing education moved from the hospital to higher education settings, the scientific and humanistic aspects of nursing were again emphasized. For example, when Yale established its school of nursing, the curriculum was designed to provide a scientific background with a particular focus to build nurses' skills in caring for the whole patient (Dolan, 1985). Schools of nursing required courses taken in the behavioral sciences and often emphasized the psychosocial aspects of nursing.

Even with the development of independent schools of nursing, tensions within the caring/curing context continued. While hospitals continued to emphasize the importance of curing, the academic and theoretical literature in nursing supported the importance of caring.

Since the 1950s, there has been a steady increase in attention given to the caring dimension in nursing. In 1957, for instance, Krueter attempted to distinguish between the caring and curing aspects of nursing. Kreuter associated care with a feeling of competence experienced and responded to by the extension of one self to another. Cure, on the other hand, was related to the administration of technical skills via tests, medications, and treatments.

During the 1960s, and as a result of an explosion of knowledge, theoretical discoveries, and technological innovations, nursing grew in scope and complexity. Such growth served as an impetus for recommending the baccalaureate degree as the entry practice level for nursing (Palmer, 1983). Three aspects of nursing—cure, care, and coordination—came to embody nursing functions. Also in the 1960s, Lewis identified the nursing process as a means of achieving appropriate caring functions in nursing. Lewis (1968) described the direct care functions of nursing as physical care, emotional support, and teaching. During this same period, nurse theorists recognized the interpersonal process of nursing building on the work of Peplau (1952) and Orlando (1961), who have focused on caring as a process within the nurse-patient relationship. Some years later, Bevis (1978) developed a curriculum in which caring as an interpersonal process was taught in both an undergraduate and graduate nursing program.

With the expanded role of nursing evolving in the 1970s, the caring/curing dilemma again became the subject of debate. Concerns were expressed that the expanded role of nursing placed it closer to medicine, emphasizing curing rather than caring. Yet as nurses began to practice in these expanded roles, they demonstrated that they were able to integrate both caring and curing functions, and from this new found strength they were able to develop a more collegial relationship with medicine (Bates, 1970).

In addition, new strategies for the delivery of nursing care emerged which facilitated practice in a more caring way. Some of these methods were primary nursing and community nursing clinics. Lewis and Resnik (1966), in a study on patients seen in nursing clinics, demonstrated that patients were more satisfied and more compliant than in traditional medical clinics. With the increased knowledge of nurses and the expanded role of nursing, Lysaught (1972) argued that nursing should give at least equal attention to care and wellness.

Madeleine Leininger is an academician who has promoted scholarly work on caring. Through her ethnoscience research and creation of the International Association of Human Caring, Leininger encouraged and assisted nurses to investigate caring. More specifically, through her research, Leininger developed a taxonomy of caring constructs in 30 different cultures. Leininger argues forcefully that nursing needs to develop new models of health care and different kinds of caring systems for different social, cultural, and economic groups.

Leininger (1984) proposed two realms of caring: humanistic and professional. She described humanistic caring in a generic sense as those activities which are assisting, supportive, and facilitate activities toward another. Professional nursing caring consists of those activities, cognitively learned from humanistic and scientific models, about helping individuals and groups to receive "personalized services through culturally specific or ascribed caring process, techniques, and patterns in order to improve or maintain a favorable healthy condition for life and death."

CURRENT DILEMMA RELATED TO CARING IN NURSING

Although caring has evolved as an important element of nursing practice, several factors threaten its continued central focus for nursing. Lysaught (1981), who views caring as the epitome of nursing also points out how quickly it is stifled by other demands on nursing. The increased use of technology, the bureaucratic institutional constraints, the focus of cost savings in health care, the subservience of nursing to medicine, and, at time, the lack of accountability in nursing are several pressures which threaten the placement of caring as a priority in nursing.

In the 1980s, from both education and research perspectives, caring has received more attention. Benner (1989), for example, identified caring actions in narratives by nurses. In 1988, a National League for Nursing resolution called for curricula that reflect the goal of enhancement of caring practices that are egalitarian and characterized by cooperation and community building. In this view, caring is a core value and central to nursing.

From the clinical perspective, the emphasis on caring in nursing remains threatened and at times hidden. Tanner (1990) effectively underscored the invisibility of caring by stating to educators that it is "important to make visible to our students the invisible caring practices of nurses" (p. 72). The economic concerns of health care have overshadowed humanitarian needs. Watson (1990) stated that caring as a core value cannot be forthcoming in our health care system until the system is revolutionized.

To counter consumer concerns that caring is not a high priority in the health care system, nurses, physicians, and health care administrators are becoming more aware of the importance of caring in the delivery of health care. As stated by one physician, the disenchantment that the public has with physicians "probably reflects the perceptions by people that they are not being cared for" (Eisenberg,

1977). Today more than ever, nursing faces the challenge of identifying the elements unique to nursing and of value to the consumer. If nursing can overcome some of its difficulties and constraints, it has the opportunity to assume a leadership role in fully integrating caring within the delivery of health care. To accomplish this task, nurses need to reestablish caring as a central characteristic of professional nursing and place it in a scientific perspective or they need to disassociate themselves from their previous embodiment as a profession.

CARING AS A CHARACTERISTIC OF A PROFESSION

Lysaught (1981) identified six characteristics of a full profession: (1) a strong level of commitment; (2) a long and disciplined educational process; (3) a unique body of knowledge and skills; (4) discretionary authority and judgment; (5) an active and cohesive professional organization; and (6) acknowledged social worth. Historically, the advancement of a discipline from a vocation to an occupation to a profession has been driven by three major forces: (1) the transition from a charitable to an economic base; (2) the identification of a specialized knowledge which communicates a sense of mystery; and (3) a masculine orientation. In its goal to become a full profession, nursing has been hindered by its feminine predominance and its emphasis on caring. The following analysis illustrates how caring has partially blocked nursing from achieving full professional status through its resistance to the three forces which have driven the development of professionalization in various disciplines.

FROM A CHARITABLE TO AN ECONOMIC BASE

One characteristic of a profession identified earlier by Flexner (1915) is this: it is motivated by altruism. The mission or purpose of a profession often starts from charity, being derived from a need to serve mankind in some special manner. An aspect of the first steps toward professionalization is the evolution away from the charity base toward an economic base. In this evolution, an economic base gains justification by way of an advancement toward professionalization: a profession becomes increasingly scientific and requires a specialized knowledge that results in a sophisticated educational process (Lysaught, 1981).

Medicine exemplifies this advancement. Although medicine never lost its service orientation, it became embedded in science and economics. Thus, as medicine evolved, it became less focused on caring and more focused on curing, science, and technology.

Hughes (1965) argued that one theme of professionalization is detachment or the withdrawal of personal interest toward the development of scientific interest and social controls. As a result, and as specialization increases, the professional relationship often becomes depersonalized (Gustafson, 1982). Thus, in opposition to its altruistic origins, in the process of professionalization, the professional person learns to relate to clients in an objective rather than subjective manner.

The nurse–patient relationship, which is based on the subjectivity required and a therapeutic relationship, is the cornerstone of nursing. The value of this relationship and its caring elements may have partially prevented nurses from placing this relationship in an objective perspective.

SPECIALIZED KNOWLEDGE

According to Moloney (1986), another attribute of professions is their development of a sense of mystery. This aura of mystery is created by the professions' use of specialized knowledge. With an increase in the knowledge specific to its domain, a profession develops its own terminology. The use of specialized terminology increases the mysteriousness of a profession and the social distance between the professional person and those served. One outcome of this process may be the fear of reduction of the caring dimension of the profession.

It may also be one of the reasons that caring practices of nurses are frequently invisible and understated.

Until recently, caring has not been seen as a field for scientific inquiry. Thus, there has been little professional incentive to study caring or discipline oneself to practice in a caring manner. Instead, caring was often perceived by the professional as an ideal, even aloof concept (Styles, 1982). Only since the 1980s have nurse researchers recognized caring as a legitimate area of scientific inquiry.

Jean Watson (1979, 1985) suggested that since science and humanism are both inherent in nursing, the profession should be based upon "the science of caring." Watson described science as neutral to human value and concerned with methodological procedures, accurate predictions, and comprehensive generalizations. In contrast, humanities are based on human goals and experiences and the emotional response to experiences. According to Watson, the science of caring is a blending of a scientific and humanistic approach, achieving a delicate balance between scientific methods and humanistic values. With this description, Watson argued that the science of caring is an appropriate area for study in nursing.

MASCULINE ORIENTATION

Another factor which thwarts caring is that the major or consulting professions (medicine and law) have been dominated by men. Since caring originates with maternal care, it is often seen as the domain of women. While women were placed in caretaker roles, men were to become more knowledgeable about living in the world. Nursing readily illustrates this cultural division. As an historically female profession, nursing has always been dominated by the male profession of medicine. We must remember that the professional sovereignty of American medicine was historically and culturally established (Starr, 1982). Nursing was delegated the task of taking care of patients, which permitted medicine to go on to its more important and certainly self-serving scientific work of curing patients.

Likewise, until recently nurses emulated medicine by delegating the task of direct care provider downward. However, with the advent of clinical nurse specialists and primary nursing, nursing has begun to reverse this practice and become more involved with patients by increasingly providing direct care.

CONSEQUENCES OF CARING IN THE PROFESSIONS

Because of the forces described, caring often has been considered a less important professional attribute. The evolution of a profession is not without risks both to the discipline which becomes a profession and to the persons within the profession.

An inability to be able to care for those you serve can be demoralizing to the person who is practicing his or her profession. The danger of treating others as objects is that it may perpetuate the view of self as an object. A defense against this danger is to "care for" the science or knowledge base of the profession.

In addition, the public may become disenchanted with a profession which does not embody some aspects of caring and feel hostility against the profession. Some problems that historically and currently face medicine in part, may be due to a loss of some of its caring characteristics as perceived by the public. Menninger (1975) stated that the medical profession cannot disregard consumer feedback regarding its insufficient caring qualities. Eisenberg (1977) elaborated that the cost of the Flexner model of education was the increasing discrepancy between what the physician was trained to do and what the public wanted. The public's perception of the economic affluence of physicians and their lack of caring has generated considerable hostility towards medicine.

CARING AND THE FUTURE PROFESSIONALIZATION OF NURSING

In order to promote nursing as a profession which has caring as a major element, several assumptions regarding caring are important:

1. Caring is a central and unifying dimension of nursing.*
2. Caring is essential for human growth.*
3. Caring is universally experienced.*
4. Caring is expressed differently within cultures.*
5. Caring behaviors can be learned.
6. Self caring is an antecedent to caring for others.
7. Caring is a necessary and sufficient activity that may be separate or may *not* be associated with curing.*
8. Caring can be categorized into subconstructs.*
9. Caring can be scientifically studied.*

CONCLUSIONS

Caring as a critical concept needs to be more appreciated, visible and investigated. It is the very concept that brings nursing together (Lynaugh & Fagin, 1988). In the last two decades, nursing has made progress towards professionalization, but greater strides need to be made if this goal is to be met. As nurses have progressed in this direction, some nurses have identified caring as a central core of their practice. It is not accidental or serendipitous that progress has been made in both of these two areas: caring and professionalism. The caring dimension of nursing helps to establish the independent practice area of nursing, and the growth in professionalism endows caring with a strength that did not exist when it was viewed as a "weak" form of occupational behavior. If caring is not compatible with a professional characteristic, nursing needs to question the traditional routes for professional status. On the other hand, if it is accepted that caring is essential and central to nursing, then it follows that nursing's primary attention should be focused on the practice, study, and teaching of caring within the nursing content.

---

* Leininger, M. M. (1984). *Care, the essence of nursing and health.* Thorofare, NJ: Slack.

In educating nurses, the altruistic aspect of nursing should not be shunned. Rather, it should be emphasized in nursing education in order to focus on self-care and caring for others. The physical, technical, and behavioral aspects of nursing can be taught within a caring framework to educate and socialize student nurses to view caring as a tangible rather than an abstract concept. To accomplish this, faculty will need to model the caring role in their professional relationships with students and patients. The learning of caring will be enhanced when school cultures promote caring practices and students perceive themselves as being treated with respect and with full consideration of their individual talents.

Nursing needs to demonstrate to health care administrators and physicians that the caring practices will increase the well being of patients and, thus, promote cost-effective quality care. To do this, nurses and other health care professionals will need to learn to place an economic value on caring. Nurses need to make their caring practices visible and study the effects of these practices on cost of health care. In addition, organizational models which facilitate the practice of caring need to be identified and created. Administrators will need to ask how they can provide opportunities to care for those entrusted with the provision of care to patients.

Caring needs to be a priority in nursing research. Research methodologies need to be explicated to study the many facets of caring as an art and a science. To better address research on caring, qualitative research methodologies need to be given equal emphasis as quantitative research methods.

Some research questions:

1. Determine the relationship between caring processes and activities with consumers' perceptions of quality of care.
2. Determine the relationship between caring processes and activities with cost of care.
3. Determine how working environments influence the practice of caring.
4. Determine effective strategies to teach caring.
5. Ascertain the conditions needed to be a caring-centered practitioner.

6. Identify how professional attributes will impede or enhance the caring practice of nursing.

7. Determine the decision-making process used by nurses in implementing caring strategies.

In summary, as Styles (1982) has written, if nursing's destiny is to be cast into a profession with its traditional list of characteristics, then very little has been accomplished. The challenge for nursing is to fully realize its caring dimension and, if possible, to integrate caring as an important characteristic of a full profession in twenty-first century America.

The primary challenge is to overcome current obstacles by embracing our caring dimension and then creating models for nursing which place caring at the center. The second challenge in nursing is to expand our professional attributes to include caring. In nursing's quest for professional status, it is critical that the primary purpose in our being is not lost or forgotten.

REFERENCES

Aydelotte, M. (1983). Professional nursing: The drive for governance. In N. Chaska (Ed.), *The nursing profession: Time to speak*. New York: McGraw-Hill.

Bates, B. (1970, July 16). Doctor and nurse: Changing roles and relations. *New England Journal of Medicine, 283,* 129–134.

Benner, P., & Wrubel, J. (1988). *The primacy of caring*. Menlo Park, CA: Addison-Wesley.

Bevis, E.O. (1978). *Curriculum building in nursing*. St. Louis: C. V. Mosby.

Dolan, J. (1985). *Nursing in society: A historical perspective*. Philadelphia: W. B. Saunders.

Eisenberg, L. (1977). The search of care. *Daedalus, 106,* 235–246.

Flexner, A. (1915). Is social work a profession. *Proceedings of the National Conference of Charities and Corrections*. Chicago, IL: Hildermann Printing Company, 578–581.

Gaut, D. (1983). Development of a theoretically adequate description of caring. *Western Journal of Nursing Research, 5*(4), 313–322.

Gustafson, J. (1982). Professions as "Callings." *Social Service Review,* 501–515.

Hughes, E. C. (1965). Professions. In K. S. Lynn & the Eds. of *Daedalus, The professions in America*. Boston: Houghton Mifflin.

Krueter, F. (1957). What is good nursing care? *Nursing Outlook, 5*, 302–304.

Leininger, M. M. (1984). Caring is nursing: Understanding the meaning, importance, and issue. In M. M. Leininger (Ed.), *Care: The essence of nursing and health*. Thorofare, NJ: Slack.

Lewis, C. E., & Resnik, B. A. (1966). Relative orientation of students of medicine and nursing to ambulatory patient care. *Journal of Medical Education, 41*, 162–166.

Lewis, L. (1968). This I believe about the nursing process-key to care. *Nursing Outlook, 68*, 26–29.

Lynaugh, J., & Fagin, C. (1988). Nursing comes of age. *Image, 20*(4), 184–190.

Lysaught, J. (1972). Distributive health care needs and the occupational health nurse. *Occupational Health Nursing, 7*–11.

Lysaught, J. (1981). *Action in affirmation: Toward an unambiguous profession of nursing*. New York: McGraw-Hill.

Mayeroff, M. (1971). *On caring*. New York: Harper & Row.

Menninger, W. W. (1975, November 24). Caring as part of health care quality. *Journal of the American Medical Association, 234*, 836–837.

Moloney, M. (1986). *Professionalism of nursing*. Philadelphia: J. B. Lippincott.

National league for Nursing. (1989). Resolution #12: Support for Innovative Curricula for Nursing Education (News). *Nursing in Health Care, 10*, 386.

Nightingale, F. (1964). *Notes on nursing: What it is and what it is not*. Philadelphia: J. B. Lippincott.

Orlando, I. (1961). *The dynamic nurse–patient relationship*. New York: G. P. Putman.

Palmer, I. (1983). From whence we come. In N. Chaska (Ed.), *The nursing profession: A time to speak*. New York: McGraw-Hill.

Peabody, W. (1927). The care of the patient. *Journal of the American Medical Association, 88*, 877–882.

Peplau, H. (1952). *Interpersonal relations in nursing*. New York: G. P. Putman.

Reverby, S. (1990). The duty or right to care, nursing and womanhood in historical perspective. In R. Abey & M. Nelson (Eds.), *Circles of care*. Albany, NY: State University of New York Press.

Starr, P. (1982). *The social transformation of American medicine*. New York: Basic Books.

Styles, M. (1982). *On nursing toward a new endowment*. St. Louis: C. V. Mosby.

Tanner, C. (1990). Caring as a value in nursing education. *Nursing Outlook, 38*(2), 70–72.

Watson, J. (1990). The moral failure of the patriarchy. *Nursing Outlook,* 38(2), 62–65.

Watson, J. (1979). *Nursing: The philosophy and science of caring.* Boston: Little Brown.

Watson, J. (1985). *Nursing: Human science and human care.* Norwalk, CT: Appleton-Century-Crofts.

17

The Magic of Caring

Patricia C. Ira

Nurses, like many women today, are afraid of caring. They view caring, an insight traditionally attributed to women, as an indicator of their failure to be assimilated into society's mainstream (Gordon, 1991). Current economic and political forces emphasize competition, power, and personal wealth. Those who practice caring in such an environment risk being forced into positions that are undervalued. To combat this threat, nurses need to transform society's values to caring, empowerment, and recognition of human worth. To achieve this transformation, nurses need a new model, a new heroine. In this paper, I will develop a qualitative ethnonursing research proposal for investigating how caring is demonstrated in undergraduate nursing programs and how the transmission of caring knowledge from nursing faculty to nursing students can be a model for society at large.

A brave new heroine for nurses emerges from Helgelsen's (1990) *The Female Advantage*. Historically, culture has developed a dichotomized system of viewing heros. For women, the heroic symbol was the Martyr which epitomized care, sacrifice, and suffering. For men, the Warrior epitomized individuation, achievement, and action. Helgelsen's amalgam of the qualities of both, the Magician, can become a new heroine for nurses. Her conception of the Magician moves beyond previously expressed dualities forging the qualities of both into a heroine that is enabled by an awareness of the interconnections that bind all human beings. "The Magician incorporates the Martyr's emphasis on care and serving others with the Warrior's ability to affect the environment by the exercise of discipline, struggle, and will" (p. 256). The arena of the new heroine is a circle, a figure that has been associated with magicians in all cultures. Centered in the circle the Magician accesses the world through a web of relationships with a magnetic force that can "attract and galvanize positive energy for change by identifying places where growth can occur for individuals . . . and then by fostering that growth" (p. 257).

This mythical Magician construction has a human counterpart. The figure of the circle and the force of the magnet are realized in every genuinely caring teacher-student and nurse-patient encounter. Caring is the ephemeral force that nurtures and enables growth within the circumference of the one-caring and the cared-for. While the value of caring is espoused by the discipline of nursing, seldom is it incorporated into the curricula as an organizing concept. The University of Colorado, Georgia Southern College, and Florida Atlantic University are three institutions who have set the example of organizing their curricula around the core concept of caring (Clayton & Murray, 1989). Their action reflects growing recognition of the need to study how caring knowledge is realized and transmitted for the continuation and development of the science of caring.

DOMAIN

In this study, the domain of inquiry concerns baccalaureate nursing education; specifically, that area where caring knowledge is transmitted from expert to novice nurses within classroom, clinical, and extracurricular areas. The research questions for the study include:

1. What does caring mean to the nurse educator?
2. What does caring mean to the nursing student?
3. How has the nursing student's conception of caring changed during the undergraduate experience?
4. How is caring included in the university philosophy?

The rationale for this choice is that in our rapidly changing society, educational institutions must do more than provide information; they need to "provide the tools with which one can become wise and mature" (Bevis, 1989, p. 67). Over a decade ago Leininger warned, "For survival, human development, self-actualization, and human relatedness to occur, care needs to occur" (1980, p. 143). Care, the core of nursing, is a most powerful means for the development of maturity and wisdom.

Nursing baccalaureate educational institutions are in the unique position of promoting the values of the nursing discipline as they define the nurse of the future. This advantage is lost when caring is relegated to the "illegitimate curriculum" (Bevis, 1989); that curriculum that is taught but never acknowledged on paper because of the difficulty in measuring it with behavioral objectives. The teaching of caring is left to the vagaries of the individual instructor's priorities and abilities.

The significance of the transmission of caring knowledge stems from the unique need of nursing students to "be presented the opportunity to know themselves ontologically as caring persons and professionals and to understand how caring orders their lives" (Boykin & Schoenhofer, 1991, p. 154). The ability of nursing students to care for others is rooted in their personal experience of being cared for themselves.

If nurses are to be more than technicians, more than a mass produced "product for institutions" (Watson, 1989a, p. 423) we cannot tolerate the denigration of caring. Rather, we must explicate the essence of caring and place it in its true social and ethical perspective. In our educational institutions, scholars who combine the roles of nurse-teacher-researcher are uniquely qualified by their combined expertise in the humanities, biological sciences, and research methods to play this vital role.

STUDY CONTEXT

Two landmark events related to nursing education occurred in the early years of this century. First, in 1917 the National League for Nursing published a *Standard Curriculum for Schools of Nursing* requiring the teaching institutions, mostly hospital-based apprenticeship programs, to be primarily concerned with the education of students rather than the provision of service for the hospitals. Second, in 1937 at Yale University the first collegiate nursing program to have its own budget and dean was established (Kalisch & Kalisch, 1978). Despite the diversity in their goals, diploma programs, collegiate programs, and the later developing associate degree programs adopted the Tyler (1949) model of curriculum development. This decision was probably influenced by two factors: the Tyler model was the standard used by both national and state board accreditation agencies and nurses obtaining higher degrees were obtaining them in schools of education where the Tyler model originated (Bevis, 1989).

The Tyler model is a product of the behaviorist influence in education during the 1940s. According to the Tyler model, changes in behavior are the measure of learning. Learning can be characterized by the determination of behavioral objectives, the selection and organization of learning experiences, and the evaluation of outcomes. The model has the advantages of being responsive to societal trust and of maintaining a reliable quality of graduates in the areas measured. The limits of the model center about its exclusivity: it mandates behavioral objectives for all learning. Goals that are not empirically verifiable are not addressed. That joyous part of education, "the teaching of inquiry, reflection, criticism, independence, creativity, and caring" (Bevis, 1989, p. 3), goes unrecognized, remains hidden, as to seem illegitimate.

Currently, behaviorism is not consistent with the philosophical underpinnings of nursing theories that share such themes as process, evolution of consciousness, self-transcendence, open systems, harmony, relativity of space-time, and pattern and holism (Sarter, 1988). Although such themes cannot be bound by deterministic or reductionist methods, they are reflected in the theoretic description of caring as described by Gaut (1984). In her logical conditions for caring, she includes awareness, knowledge, intention, positive change, and the welfare of the person. Awareness, for Gaut, entails personal respect for the dignity and rights of the cared-for. Knowledge is understanding the other's need and responding to those needs. The intention for positive change involves recognizing that the action chosen is based solely on the welfare of the other. Each of these conditions is a holistic process that requires openness and the ability to transcend self. Each evolves over time and displays a characteristic pattern.

The philosophy of the present research rests on the following major assumptions concerning the transmission of caring knowledge: (1) care is essential for human growth and development; (2) care is the moral imperative of nursing and nursing education; (3) care knowledge can be transmitted; (4) a caring teacher-student interaction is a prerequisite for a caring student-patient interaction; and (5) the culture of the nursing education institution influences the student's perception of the value of caring.

The ontological dimension of care, or care in itself, is expressed in Roach's (1991) conceptualization of caring as "a human mode of being . . . an expression of our humanity, essential to our development and fulfillment as human beings" (p. 8). The idea of fulfillment is echoed in Nouwen's (1978) description of the redemptive process that is the essential relationship between the teacher and learner. Nouwen characterizes the process as: (1) evocative in that each is available to the other, (2) bilateral in that each participant is willing to be influenced by the other, and (3) actualizing in that learning not only prepares for the future but also becomes actuated in the present. Thus a mutual enabling of individual potential is evoked through the consciousness of the other. Nouwen posits that "we have paid too much attention to the content of teaching without realizing that the teaching relationship is the most important function in the ministry of teaching" (p. 5).

What is the state of the teaching relationship in caring science? How do novice nurses come to know caring? Belenky, Clinchy, Goldberger, and Tarule (1986) studied women's ways of knowing and developed a framework which identifies the five patterns that emerge: (1) silence in which abstract thought is underdeveloped and the dictates of authority are accepted; (2) received knowledge in which the ability to receive and reproduce knowledge is employed but knowledge development is viewed as dependent on others; (3) subjective knowledge in which the private inner voice is used by the individual but not appraised or articulated; (4) procedural knowledge in which the individual objectively observes, systematically analyzes and structures what is known; and (5) constructed knowledge in which a pattern dependent on context inclusive of objective and subjective experience integrates all previous ways of knowing. Throughout academic and clinical experiences the sensitive nurse educator enables students to identify their own patterns of knowing within this framework and generates the positive energy needed for growth to occur.

Noddings (1984) prioritizes the role of the teacher in transmitting knowledge of human caring. In professions such as nursing where encounter is frequent, the teacher is first and foremost one-caring and only secondarily a teacher or a nurse. "The student is infinitely more important than the subject matter" (p. 176). To be totally and nonselectively present to the student, to each student (p. 180) is necessary in promoting the ethical ideal of caring. This is accomplished through the activities of modeling, dialogue, practice, and confirmation.

Watson (1989b) discusses the need for "transpersonal caring contacts between students and faculty" (p. 57) using Nodding's four activities. The mutuality of the activities is apparent in her description. Mutual growth is accomplished by modeling caring in action. Taking advantage of teaching moments and using them as "caring occasions" promotes mutual self-discovery. Genuine dialogue where caring is expressed openly aids in the mutual search for enlightenment. In the practice situation, students are not only cared for and supported by the teacher but also encouraged to care for and support each other. They are encouraged and shown how to care for themselves by recognizing and dealing with the stress inherent in their situation. Confirmation is seen as a powerful formative force in the development of human consciousness. According to Watson, "it is here in our educational caring occasion where we lay the very foundation for human caring in health care; we lay the very foundation for creating a context of community for, and of, caring" (p. 57).

Explicating how caring knowledge is transmitted in nursing education enables nursing educators to help their students recognize the unique qualities of women's ways of knowing and to make maximal use of the caring occasion to promote the ethical ideal of caring. The caring way by which the educator teaches will influence the caring way by which the student practices.

LITERATURE REVIEW

There are few studies that have examined the teacher-student interaction or have focused on the caring aspect of that relationship and its effect on the future practice of the nursing student. A national survey was sent to 450 nursing baccalaureate program directors asking them if caring was taught in the curriculum and if faculty caring skills were addressed (Slevin & Harter, 1987). Of the 273 (60.7%) who responded, 70.7 percent reported caring as integrated into the curriculum, 18.1 percent reported it as a component of another concept, 6.3 percent reported it as a major concept, and 2.2 percent reported it as an organizing concept. Four problems are highlighted by this study: (1) in most programs faculty caring skills are not evaluated, (2) caring content is concentrated at the higher levels, (3) caring is seldom an organizing concept, and (4) student's perceptions of what is taught about caring are not included.

Halldorsdottir (1990) included the perceptions of nursing students who studied the essential structure of a caring encounter between students and faculty. In this phenomenological study, Halldorsdottir examined 16 in-depth, open-ended interviews regarding nine former nursing students' perceptions of caring and uncaring encounters. She found that a caring encounter had the following elements: (1) the teacher's professional caring approach which included competence, genuine concern for the student, an overall positive personality and professional commitment; and (2) mutual trust. The attributes of a positive personality included personal integrity, sharing of self, attentiveness, flexibility, and humor. The uncaring encounter was characterized by absence of competence and concern and a demand for control and other forms of destructive behavior.

A professional teacher-student working relationship was developed from the data. According to Halldorsdottir (1990), this process consists of six phases: (1) initiating attachment, (2) mutual acknowledgment of personhood, (3) development of boundaries of the working relationship, (4) negotiation of learning outcomes, (5) understanding and (6) termination. The positive outcomes observed from caring encounters include a sense of acceptance and self-worth of the student coupled with personal as well as professional growth. The effects of non-caring encounters are marked by disbelief, resentment, anger, and long-term negative feelings and memories. Halldorsdottir's study describes the meaning that teacher-student encounters have for nursing students. It gives the nursing instructor information that can assist in improving how they relate to students and how to make caring an integral part of each teaching encounter.

Appleton (1990) developed a model of pedagogical caring in a phenomenological study regarding the meaning of human care and the experience of caring in a university school of nursing. She interviewed two doctoral students. Four caring themes emerged: treating with respect, understanding independence, helping to grow, and letting become. The meaning of caring was viewed in the following contexts: personal, relational, situational, and environmental. In reformulating nursing education, Appleton considered these aspects as essential: (1) a person-oriented approach; (2) freedom to be who one is; (3) time to understand and reflect during the educational process; (4) opportunity for dialog; and (5) caring faculty who communicate clearly, criticize constructively, and confirm the student.

Griffith and Bakanauskas (cited in Murray, 1989) studied the student-teacher relationship and the use of therapeutic communication. The student's ability to learn communication skills and use them with the client was improved when teachers met the student's learning needs for trust and support. "Caring attitudes, demonstrated by an admired, respected instructor who acknowledges students' strengths and weaknesses, are significant to students' lives and their learning" (p. 194).

The significance of the teacher who inspires students and who reaches out to learn with them was highlighted in Bush's (1988) study of the characteristics of a caring nurse-teacher. A survey of 14 nursing doctoral students and an extensive review of general educational literature generated 143 characteristics which were categorized within six major concepts: "spirituality, presence, mutual respect, sensitivity, communion with the other, and organization of teaching-learning" (p. 178). A theoretical framework for teaching practice was designed to assist teachers to develop their self-awareness and to become exemplars of care "through actions, modes of reflection, and personal writing" (p. 185).

Ethnonursing is a rich theoretical research perspective that has not been used to explicate the meaning of the caring relationship between nursing students and faculty. Ethnonursing offers a most appropriate method here because of these factors: (1) it is useful in situations where little knowledge is available, (2) it elicits a totality of information, (3) it is holistic and congruent with the values of nursing, and (4) its goal is nursing knowledge. According to Leininger (1985), ethnonursing is "the systematic study and analysis of the local and indigenous people's viewpoints, beliefs, and practices about nursing care phenomena and processes of designated cultures" (p. 38).

Preliminary findings from an ethnonursing study could be used by nurse educators to assist them in planning curriculum changes in their institutions that are more consistent with the moral imperative of caring. They could be used by individual teachers to become more sensitive to students' needs and to use the teaching occasion to display caring.

CONCLUSION

Women, in particular nurses, must shed their fear of caring. Rather than hiding their ability to care, they need to study the qualities of Helgelsen's heroic Magician construction and galvanize their abilities to create a society that values human caring. Nurse scholars need to scrutinize the ephemeral force of caring and its ability to nurture and enable human growth in the bright light of systematic research. A qualitative ethnonursing research study has been proposed to examine the interconnection between the one-caring and the one-cared-for enclosed within the circumference of the teaching-learning environment and the effect it has on the transmission of caring knowledge to future generations of nurses.

REFERENCES

Appleton, C. (1990). The meaning of human care and the experience of caring in a university school of nursing. In M. M. Leininger & J. Watson (Eds.), *The caring imperative in education*. New York: National League for Nursing.

Belenky, M., Clinchy, B., Goldberger, N., & Tarule, J. (1986). *Women's ways of knowing, the development of self, voice, and mind*. New York: Basic Books.

Bevis, E. M. (1989). Nursing curriculum as professional education: Some underlying theoretical models. In E. M. Bevis & J. Watson (Eds.), *Toward a caring curriculum: A new pedagogy for nursing*. New York: National League for Nursing.

Boykin, A., & Schoenhofer, S. (1991). Caring in nursing: Analysis of extant theory. *Nursing Science Quarterly, 4*(3), 149–155.

Bush, H. A. (1988). The caring teacher of nursing. In M. M. Leininger (Ed.), *Care: Discovery and uses in clinical and community nursing*. Detroit: Wayne State University Press.

Clayton, G. M., & Murray, J. P. (1989). Faculty-student relationships: Catalytic connection. In E. O. Bevis (Ed.), *Curriculum revolution: Reconceptualizing Nursing Education*. New York: National League for Nursing.

Gaut, D. (1984). A theoretic description of caring as action. In M. M. Leininger (Ed.), *Caring: The essence of nursing and health*. Detroit: Wayne State University Press.

Gordon, S. (1991). Fear of caring: The feminist paradox. *American Journal of Nursing*, (2), 45–48.

Halldorsdottir, S. (1990). The essential structure of a caring and uncaring encounter with a teacher: The perspective of the nursing student. In M. M. Leininger & J. Watson (Eds.), *The caring imperative in education*. New York: National League for Nursing.

Helgelsen, S. (1990). *The female advantage*. New York: Doubleday & Company.

Kalish, P. A., & Kalish, B. J. (1978). *The advance of American Nursing*. Boston: Little, Brown and Company.

Leininger, M. M. (1980). Caring: A central focus of nursing and health care services. *Nursing and Health Care, 1*(3), 135–143.

Leininger, M. M. (1985). Ethnography and ethnonursing: Models and modes of qualitative data analysis. In M. M. Leininger (Ed.), *Qualitative research methods in nursing*. Orlando, FL: Grune & Stratton.

Murray, J. (1989). Making the connection: Teacher-student interactions and learning experiences. In E. M. Bevis & J. Watson (Eds.), *Toward a caring curriculum: A new pedagogy for nursing.* New York: National League for Nursing.

Nelms, T. (1990). The lived experience of nursing education: A phenomenological study. In M. M. Leininger & J. Watson (Eds.), *The caring imperative in education.* New York: National League for Nursing.

Noddings, N. (1948). *Caring: A feminine approach to ethics and moral education.* Los Angeles: University of California Press.

Nouwen, H. J. M. (1978). *Creative ministry.* Garden City, NY: Doubleday & Company.

Roach, S. (1991). The call to consciousness: Compassion in today's health world. In D. A. Gaut & M. M. Leininger (Eds.), *Caring: The compassionate healer.* Detroit: Wayne State University Press.

Sarter, B. (1988). Philosophical sources of nursing theory. *Nursing Science Quarterly, 1*(2), 52–59.

Slevin, A. P., & Harter, M. O. (1987). The teaching of caring: A survey report. *Nurse Educator, 12*(6), 23–26.

Tyler, R. (1949). *Basic principles of curriculum and instruction.* Chicago: University of Chicago Press.

Watson, J. (1989a). Human caring as moral context for nursing education. *Nursing and Health Care, 9*(8), 423–425.

Watson, J. (1989b). Transformative thinking and a caring curriculum. In E. M. Bevis & J. Watson (Eds.), *Toward a caring curriculum: A new pedagogy for nursing.* New York: National League for Nursing.